On-Field Evaluation and Treatment of
# COMMON ATHLETIC
# INJURIES

# On-Field Evaluation and Treatment of
# COMMON ATHLETIC
# INJURIES

EDITORS

## James R. Andrews, M.D.
## William G. Clancy, Jr., M.D.
## James A. Whiteside, M.D.

*with 84 illustrations*

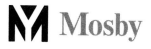

St. Louis  Baltimore  Boston  Carlsbad  Chicago  Naples  New York  Philadelphia  Portland
London  Madrid  Mexico City  Singapore  Sydney  Tokyo  Toronto  Wiesbaden

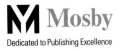
**Mosby**
Dedicated to Publishing Excellence

**A Times Mirror**
**Company**

*Vice President and Publisher:* Anne S. Patterson
*Editor:* Robert Hurley
*Developmental Editor:* Lauranne Billus
*Editorial Assistant:* Mia Cariño
*Project Manager:* Linda Clarke
*Production Editor:* Kathleen Hillock
*Composition Specialist:* Pamela Merritt
*Designer:* Carolyn O'Brien
*Manufacturing Manager:* William A. Winneberger, Jr.

**Copyright © 1997 by Mosby–Year Book, Inc.**

Printed in the United States of America
Composition by Mosby Electronic Production, Philadelphia
Printing/binding by R. R. Donnelley & Sons Co.

Mosby–Year Book, Inc.
11830 Westline Industrial Drive
St. Louis, Missouri 63146

**Library of Congress Cataloging-in-Publication Data**

On-field evaluation and treatment of common athletic injuries / James
    R. Andrews, William G. Clancy, Jr., James A. Whiteside.
            p.  cm.
        Includes index.
        ISBN 0-8151-0218-6
        1. Sports injuries. 2. First aid in illness and injury.
    I. Andrews, James R. (James Rheuben). II. Clancy, William
    G. III. Whiteside, James A.
            [DNLM: 1. Athletic Injuries—diagnosis. 2. Athletic Injuries—
            therapy. 3. First Aid. 4. Sports Medicine. WA 292 058 1997]
    RD97.04  1997
    617.1'027—dc21
    DNLM/DLC
    for Library of Congress                                              96-49798
                                                                              CIP

    98 99 00 01 / 9 8 7 6 5 4 3 2

# Editors

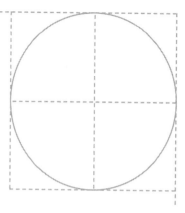

**James R. Andrews, M.D.**
Clinical Professor of Orthopaedics and
    Sports Medicine,
University of Virginia Medical School,
Charlottesville, Virginia;
Clinical Professor, Department of
    Orthopaedic Surgery,
University of Kentucky Medical Center,
Lexington, Kentucky;
Medical Director, Tampa Bay Devil Rays
    Professional Baseball Team,
Tampa Bay, Florida;
Orthopaedic Consultant, Toronto Blue Jays
    Professional Baseball Team,
Toronto, Ontario;
Senior Orthopaedic Consultant, Cincinnati
    Reds Professional Baseball Team,
Cincinnati, Ohio;
Clinical Professor of Surgery,
Division of Orthopaedic Surgery,
    Department of Surgery, School of
    Medicine,
University of Alabama at Birmingham;
Medical Director, American Sports
    Medicine Institute;
Orthopaedic Surgeon, Alabama Sports
    Medicine & Orthopaedic Center,
Birmingham, Alabama

**William G. Clancy, Jr., M.D.**
Clinical Professor of Orthopaedics and
    Sports Medicine,
University of Virginia Medical School,
Charlottesville, Virginia;
Clinical Professor of Surgery,
Division of Orthopaedic Surgery,
    Department of Surgery, School of
    Medicine,
University of Alabama at Birmingham;
Staff Orthopaedic Surgeon,
Alabama Sports Medicine & Orthopaedic
    Center,
Birmingham, Alabama

**James A. Whiteside, M.D.**
Eminent Scholar in Sports Medicine;
Clinical Associate Professor of
    Orthopaedics and Sports Medicine,
University of Virginia Medical School,
Charlottesville, Virginia;
Professor, College of Health and Human
    Services,
Team Physician,
Troy State University,
Troy, Alabama;
Staff, Nonoperative,
Alabama Sports Medicine & Orthopaedic
    Center,
Birmingham, Alabama

# Contributors

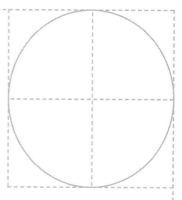

**Emory J. Alexander, M.D.**
Orthopaedic Surgeon, Spine Specialist,
Hughston Clinic, P.C.,
Columbus, Georgia

**Kenneth W. Bramlett, M.D.**
Orthopaedic Surgeon,
Alabama Sports Medicine & Orthopaedic
    Center;
Clinical Instructor,
University of Alabama at Birmingham,
Birmingham, Alabama

**Raymond J. Browne, M.D.**
Internal Medicine Consultant,
American Sports Medicine Institute and
HealthSouth Medical Center,
Birmingham, Alabama

**J. Markus Carter, D.O.**
Director of Nonsurgical Spine Care for
    Southeast Spine Surgery,
Alabama Sports Medicine & Orthopaedic
    Center,
Birmingham, Alabama

**C. Barry Craythorne, M.D.**
Orthopaedic Surgeon,
Tampa Bay Orthopaedics,
Tampa Bay, Florida

**Ronald G. Derr, D.O.**
Orthopaedic Surgeon,
The Bone and Joint Clinic,
Franklin, Tennessee

**Scott Deuel, M.S., P.T.**
Assistant Clinic Director,
Gadsden Rehabilitation Center,
Gadsden, Alabama

**Kimberly Morris Fagan, M.D.**
Clinical Instructor of Medicine,
University of Alabama at Birmingham;
Director of Medical Aspects of Sports
    Medicine,
American Sports Medicine Institute;
Physician,
Alabama Sports Medicine & Orthopaedic
    Center,
Birmingham, Alabama

**J. Stanford Faulkner, Jr., M.D.**
Orthopaedic Surgeon,
Alabama Sports Medicine & Orthopaedic
    Center,
Birmingham, Alabama

**Mark Hutchens, M.D.**
Director, Athletic Medicine,
University of Texas at Austin,
Austin, Texas;
Assistant Clinical Professor, Family Practice,
University of Texas Health Science Center,
San Antonio, Texas

**Gregg Kaiser, M.D.**
Retina and Vitreous Associates of Alabama;
Clinical Instructor, Department of
    Ophthalmology,
University of Alabama at Birmingham/Eye
    Foundation Hospital,
Birmingham, Alabama

**Michael J. Kaplan, M.D.**
Clinical Instructor, Department of
    Orthopaedics,
Yale University Medical School,
New Haven, Connecticut;
Attending Clinical Instructor,
Team Physician,
Teikyo Post University;
Director, Central Connecticut Sports
    Medicine Center,
Waterbury, Connecticut

**Ferenc Kuhn, M.D.**
Associate Professor of Clinical
    Ophthalmology,
Department of Ophthalmology,
University of Alabama at Birmingham/Eye
    Foundation Hospital;
Director of Research, United States Eye
    Injury Registry;
Associate Director of Clinical Research,
    Helen Keller Eye Research Foundation,
Birmingham, Alabama

**Scott David Martin, M.D.**
Clinical Instructor, Orthopaedic Surgery,
Harvard Medical School,
Brigham and Women's Hospital,
Boston, Massachusetts

**Keith Meister, M.D.**
Assistant Professor,
Team Physician,
University of Florida,
Shands Clinic at Hampton Oaks,
Gainesville, Florida

**Robert Morris, M.D.**
Associate Professor of Clinical
    Ophthalmology,
Department of Ophthalmology,
University of Alabama at Birmingham/Eye
    Foundation Hospital;
Founder, United States Eye Injury Registry;
President, Helen Keller Eye Research
    Foundation,
Birmingham, Alabama

**Alan G. Posta, Jr., M.D.**
Orthopaedic Surgeon,
Carolina Orthopaedic Center,
Greenville, South Carolina

**Michael A. Sclafani, M.D.**
Associate Professor,
Jersey Shore Medical Center;
Head of Sports Medicine,
Orthopaedic Institute of Central Jersey,
Sea Girt, New Jersey

**Timothy B. Sutherland, M.D.**
Clinical Instructor,
School of Medicine,
University of California–Davis,
Davis, California;
Orthopaedic Surgeon,
Desert Orthopaedic Center,
Las Vegas, Nevada

**Laura A. Timmerman, M.D.**
Associate Clinical Professor, Department of
    Orthopaedics, School of Medicine,
University of California–Davis,
Davis, California;
Team Physician,
University of California–Berkeley,
Berkley, California;
Chief of Orthopaedics,
Merrithew Hospital,
Martinez, California

**Andrew M. Tucker, M.D.**
Assistant Professor,
Department of Family Medicine,
University of Maryland School of Medicine;
Director, Primary Care Sports Medicine,
University of Maryland Medical System,
Baltimore, Maryland

**Debra S. Williams, M.D.**
Primary Care Sports Medicine,
Panama City, Florida

**John F. Wisniewski, M.S., D.M.D., F.A.C.S.M.**
Associate Professor of Dentistry,
Department of General and Hospital
    Dentistry,
University of Medicine and Dentistry of
    New Jersey—New Jersey Dental School;
Private Practice, Center for Dental and
    Oral Health,
Newark, New Jersey;
Dental Consultant to Atlanta Braves
    Professional Baseball Team,
Atlanta, Georgia;
Dental Educational Consultant to Florida
    Marlins, Houston Astros, and Kansas
    City Royals Professional Baseball Teams

**C. Douglas Witherspoon, M.D.**
Associate Professor of Clinical
    Ophthalmology,
Department of Ophthalmology,
University of Alabama at Birmingham/Eye
    Foundation Hospital;
Director, Department of Ophthalmology,
HealthSouth Medical Center;
Executive Vice President, United States Eye
    Injury Registry;
Director of Clinical Research, Helen Keller
    Eye Research Foundation;
Sports Vision Associates,
Birmingham, Alabama

# Preface

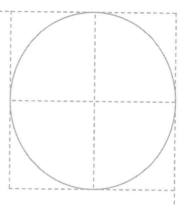

In the preface to the third edition of *Treatment of Injuries to Athletes*, published in 1976, Dr. O'Donoghue stakes no claim to originality of the information presented; rather, he emphasizes that it is the application of effective care to the injured athlete that is important. That thought is the primary precept of this book.

It is accepted that the athlete is a special person. The injured athlete must be considered as unique and deserves to be cared for in a proficient, diligent, and expedient manner. Being a skillful and knowledgeable surgeon or any equally astute medical practitioner usually does not fully prepare the person who, in an official capacity, is thrust into serving as the primary health care provider at an athletic competition.

At the Alabama Sports Medicine & Orthopaedic Center, each orthopedic and primary care sports medicine fellow is given the opportunity to care for the athletes at a local high school and one of 11 colleges and universities. These erudite and extremely well-trained fellows expressed concern that they needed more information to care for athletic types of problems adequately. In spite of twice-a-week, in-house lectures on illness, injury pattern, treatment, and rehabilitation, these young physicians proposed that a clinically based text be prepared that would describe a practical application of the current knowledge of sports medicine. That petition was the impetus that spawned the collection of articles for this book.

Of the 19 chapters, only four were written by physicians who had not experienced a sports medicine fellowship. The three section editors conferred with each author and sanctioned the written material and approved of its veracity. Except for the chapters on exercise-induced bronchospasm, heat problems, and soft tissue injuries, the other chapters deal with major anatomic sites. Considerable emphasis is given to head and neck and upper extremity injuries.

Individual chapters have been written to reveal a general appraisal of the subject matter rather than an exhaustive dissertation. The material presented should yield a workable understanding of the problems, and the care for such problems, that athletes are prone to encounter.

Those primary health care providers who cover athletic events (athletic trainers, emergency medical technicians, physician assistants, nurse practitioners, and team physicians) would profit from reflecting on and then applying the material presented in the easy-to-read text. The fundamental purpose of this book is not to replace tomes like Nicholas and Hershman's volumes on the upper and lower extremities; rather, the intent is to serve as a practical induction into properly caring for the special athlete who competes at any level.

James R. Andrews
William G. Clancy, Jr.
James A. Whiteside

## Acknowledgments

To Mrs. Jerry Conner and Mr. Dale Baker, for preparing and ramrodding the manuscripts;

To the staffs at the Alabama Sports Medicine & Orthopaedic Center and the American Sports Medicine Institute, for support; and

To past and present orthopedic and primary care sports medicine fellows, for dedication:

Our sincere appreciation and gratitude.

# Contents

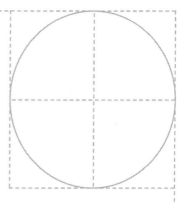

On-Field Evaluation and Treatment of
# COMMON ATHLETIC
# INJURIES

# Chapter 1

# Head and neck injuries

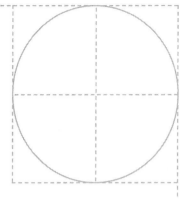

Kimberly Morris Fagan

Head and neck injuries are among the most feared of all injuries sustained in sports. The vast majority of these are minor; however, the potential for catastrophic injuries is ever present. A well-thought-out management plan can prevent a seemingly minor injury from becoming a life-threatening emergency.

## HEAD INJURIES

Head injuries range from minor concussions to permanently disabling or fatal intracranial hemorrhages. Fortunately, most head injuries are minor, and full recovery is the norm.

### CONCUSSION

A concussion—a clinical syndrome that is due to mechanical forces characterized by immediate and transient impairment of neural functions—is the most commonly occurring head injury in sports. The typical mechanism of injury involves a collision that results from an acceleration-deceleration force.

There is no general consensus on concussions. The two most frequently used guidelines vary significantly in both the grading and management of concussions in the athlete (Tables 1 and 2). However, these are only guidelines. They do not replace clinical judgement. Individualization of care is mandatory. Regardless of the classification system used, there are basic management issues to which one should adhere when caring for an athlete with a head injury.

As with any medical problem, the first step in management is recognition of the problem. Moderate to severe concussions represent little diagnostic challenge. The patient has a significant degree of amnesia and/or has loss of consciousness. The grade I concussion can easily go

**Table 1**
**EXAMPLES OF DIFFERING CONCUSSION CLASSIFICATION SYSTEMS AND RETURN-TO-PLAY RECOMMENDATIONS**

| Guidelines of | Severity | | |
| --- | --- | --- | --- |
| | Grade I (mild) | Grade II (moderate) | Grade III (severe) |
| Robert C. Cantu, M.D. | No LOC<br>Posttraumatic amnesia < 30 min | LOC < 5 min<br>Posttraumatic amnesia > 30 min | LOC > 5 min<br>Posttraumatic amnesia > 24 hr |
| The Colorado Medical Society | Confusion with amnesia<br>No LOC | Confusion with amnesia<br>No LOC | LOC |

*LOC,* Loss of consciousness.

**Table 2**
**RETURN-TO-PLAY RECOMMENDATIONS**

| | First concussion | Second concussion | Third concussion |
|---|---|---|---|
| **Guidelines of Robert C. Cantu, M.D.** | | | |
| Grade I (Mild) | May return to play if asymptomatic | May return in 2 wk if asymptomatic at that time for 1 wk | Terminate season<br>May return next yr if asymptomatic |
| Grade II (Moderate) | Return after asymptomatic for 1 wk | Wait at least 1 mo<br>May return then if asymptomatic for 1 wk<br>Consider terminating season | Terminate season<br>May return next yr if asymptomatic |
| Grade III (Severe) | Wait at least 1 mo<br>May return then if asymptomatic for 1 wk | Terminate season<br>May return next yr if asymptomatic | |
| **Guidelines of the Colorado Medical Society** | | | |
| Grade I (Mild) | May return to play if asymptomatic for at least 20 min | Terminate contest or practice for the day | Terminate season<br>May return in 3 mo if asymptomatic |
| Grade II (Moderate) | Terminate contest or practice<br>May return if asymptomatic for at least 1 wk | Consider terminating season<br>May return if asymptomatic for 1 mo | Terminate season<br>May return next season if asymptomatic |
| Grade III (Severe) | May return after 1 mo if asymptomatic for 2 wk at that time<br>May resume conditioning sooner if asymptomatic for 2 wk | Terminate season<br>Discourage any return to contact sports | |

undiagnosed. The player may not report being "dinged" and will continue to play. It is frequently a fellow athlete who reports that the injured player is "acting weird."

Once recognition has been established, a complete evaluation follows. (See the box below.) All athletes who suffer a head injury require at least temporary removal from the game. A grade I concussion requires a thorough sideline neurologic evaluation. Orientation to person, place, and time is established. Recall of events preceding and following the injury is noted. Coordination is evaluated with finger-to-nose, heel-to-shin, and Romberg's testing. Sideline agility tests are also useful. Complaints of headache, dizziness, and nausea, and signs of impaired concentration should be taken seriously. Any focal signs of motor or sensory dysfunc-

**HEAD INJURY EXAM CHECKLIST**

Rule out cervical spine injury
Rule out skull fractures or lacerations
Mental status assessment
  Alert and oriented × 3
  Normal speech
  Appropriate responses
  Intact memory (before and after injury)
Cranial nerves
  Equal pupils
  Intact light response
  Intact extraocular muscles
  Normal visual fields
  Symmetrical facial sensation and movement
  Intact hearing (whisper test)
  Intact gag reflex
Motor–sensory
  Normal muscle tone
  Normal muscle strength
  Intact light touch
  Normal deep tendon reflexes
  Negative Romberg's test
  Normal finger to nose testing
  Normal rapid alternating movements
Do not rush the exam!

tion, as well as pupil inequality, should alert one to the need for further evaluation.

If all tests are normal, the player should be observed on the sideline for a period of time. Reevaluation before return to play is mandatory. After return to play has occurred, continued observation of the athlete is necessary to detect any subtle changes in reaction time, coordination, or concentration.

In moderate to severe concussions, management differs based on the level of consciousness. The unconscious player is treated as having a cervical spine injury until proven otherwise. The basics of cardiopulmonary resuscitation (CPR)—airway, breathing, and circulation—are addressed first and foremost. After cardiorespiratory problems are handled the athlete is transported to the sideline on a fracture board, with care taken to stabilize the head and neck. A neurologic evaluation guided by the Glasgow Coma Scale is documented if time permits (Table 3).

**Table 3**
**THE GLASGOW COMA SCALE**

| Response | Points |
| --- | --- |
| **Eye opening** | |
| Spontaneous | 4 |
| To verbal command | 3 |
| To pain | 2 |
| None | 1 |
| **Best motor response** | |
| Obeys verbal command | 6 |
| Localizes pain | 5 |
| Withdraws from pain | 4 |
| Decorticate posturing | 3 |
| Decerebrate posturing | 2 |
| No response | 1 |
| **Best verbal response** | |
| Oriented and converses | 5 |
| Disoriented and converses | 4 |
| Inappropriate words | 3 |
| Incomprehensible sounds | 2 |
| No response | 1 |
| **SCORE** | **3-15** |

Transportation to a medical center—preferably one with computed tomography (CT), magnetic resonance imaging (MRI), and neurosurgical consultation available—is accomplished as soon as possible. If transport time is prolonged or transfer delayed, parenteral corticosteroids should be considered. Methylprednisolone (15 to 30 mg/kg) or dexamethasone (3 to 6 mg/kg) is suggested with the hope of preventing or modulating the effects of increased intracranial pressure. Further evaluation includes cervical spine films and a CT scan of the head. Hospitalization for further treatment or evaluation may be necessary.

In less severe cases, where unconsciousness is brief and the player is responsive, removal on a fracture board may not be necessary. However, further neurologic evaluation at an appropriate facility is recommended.

As previously stated, a clear consensus for return to play following a concussion is not well established. A general guideline (Table 2) is helpful, but individualization is necessary. This should be based on the individual player's neurologic exam, mental status, grade of concussion, previous history of concussions, and the sport involved. Charts do not replace clinical judgement. Be prudent, and "When in doubt, keep them out."

The majority of concussions resolve without sequelae. There are, however, concerns over the possibility of postconcussion syndrome and second impact syndrome. The postconcussion syndrome—which consists of headaches, fatigue, irritability, and impaired memory and concentration—is believed to be due to altered neurotransmitter function. Correlation between the duration of posttraumatic amnesia and postconcussion syndrome has been noted. Persistence of these symptoms should eliminate the athlete from play and require further evaluation that includes neuropsychiatric testing and a CT scan or MRI.

The second impact syndrome is more serious and can lead to a fatal outcome. As first described by Schneider, this is an entity in which a relatively minor blow to the head following an initial concussion produces potentially fatal brain swelling. Those at risk are felt to be the athletes with residual symptoms such as headaches, dizziness, or memory or concentration deficits. It is imperative that an athlete who does not follow the expected course of recovery undergo complete neurologic evaluation by knowledgeable physicians and with appropriate tests. Participation in sports should not be allowed as long as symptoms persist at rest or with exertion.

## INTRACRANIAL HEMORRHAGES

One of the major concerns when evaluating an athlete with a head injury is the possibility of a potentially fatal intracranial bleed. It is important to be alert to the signs and symptoms that suggest possibly more than a concussion:

- Increasing headache
- Nausea or vomiting
- Pupil irregularity
- Localizing neurologic deficits
- Confusion
- Progressive impairment of consciousness
- Sudden unconsciousness
- Rising blood pressure
- Falling pulse rate

An epidural hematoma can occur in an athlete who takes a hard blow to the head. It is typically (90% of the time) associated with a skull fracture. A tear of a meningeal artery is the usual source of bleeding. The classic presentation is an immediate loss of consciousness followed by a "lucid interval." Subsequent deterioration of mental status occurs. Some patients, however, never lose consciousness, and others never regain it after initial loss of consciousness.

Prognosis is highly dependent on the timeliness of appropriate intervention. A high index of suspicion should be maintained with all head injuries.

Subdural hematomas also occur as the result of head trauma. These involve tears of the bridging veins between the cavernous sinus and the brain. Presentation is variable. Classically the patient is initially conscious with deterioration of mental status over the next few hours to days. Mortality resulting from a subdural hematoma is in part dependent on the promptness of appropriate surgical intervention. More significantly, it is dependent on any associated cortical or brain stem damage. Therefore, unconsciousness and localizing neurologic signs noted at the time of hospital admission portend a worse outcome.

Because of the possibility of delayed neurologic decompensation it is important that athletes with head injuries, especially those rendered unconscious, be closely observed for at least a 24-hour period. Any persistence of symptoms previously mentioned or any change in neurologic status warrants a CT scan to rule out intracranial hemorrhage.

## NECK INJURIES

Neck injuries, like head injuries, range from insignificant to catastrophic. The most common types of injury are strains and sprains. The most critical are unstable cervical spine injuries with or without associated fractures. An organized approach to the diagnosis and treatment of these injuries is crucial.

## BURNER SYNDROME

Brachial plexus injuries with their associated neurologic signs and symptoms can mimic cervical spine injuries. The mechanism of injury is typically ipsilateral shoulder depression with lateral neck deviation to the contralateral side. A traction injury to the upper trunk (nerve roots C5 and C6) of the brachial plexus results. The corresponding clinical presentation is referred to as the burner syndrome.

The burner syndrome or "stinger" is one of the most common injuries in football. It typically presents as a burning pain or numbness about the shoulder. Radiation down the arm gives a "dead arm" sensation. Weakness of the involved extremity is common. Bilateral upper extremity involvement or any involvement of the lower extremity is not consistent with the diagnosis of burner syndrome.

Sideline evaluation includes palpation of the cervical spine and cervical range of motion testing. A complete cervical neurologic exam is performed. Arm weakness with associated decreased sensation is expected. Any cervical tenderness or limited or painful cervical range of motion alerts one to a more serious problem involving the cervical spine. This is true even if the cervical neurologic exam is normal.

Treatment of the typical burner syndrome includes observation and serial evaluations. Recovery is generally within minutes. Once full strength has returned and all neurologic signs and symptoms have resolved, return to play is allowed. More prolonged (hours to weeks) or recurrent episodes mandate further evaluation by a physician.

Complete evaluation of prolonged or recurrent burner syndrome is recommended to rule out cervical instability or cervical stenosis. At the minimum, cervical spine roentgenograms are obtained. These include anteroposterior (AP), lateral, and oblique views. The odontoid view is included if neck discomfort is noted at a higher level. If normal, then lateral views in flexion-extension are performed to identify subtle ligamentous instability. Assessment for cervical stenosis is also included. The Torg ratio is often used for this evaluation. This is obtained by taking the ratio of the vertebral canal width to that of the vertebral body width at approximately C4 on the lateral cervical spine film. A ratio of less than 0.8 is believed by some to be significant. Of note is a study by Oder et al, which found that of 224 football players, approximately one third had ratios of less than 0.8. This suggests that more sophisticated studies such as MRI are necessary to appropriately advise those athletes believed to be at increased risk for cervical stenosis.

In an effort to prevent this traction injury to the brachial plexus a neck strengthening program is advised. Properly fitted shoulder pads are essential. Additional posterior and lateral support such as provided with a Cowboy collar may be helpful. Educating the player about appropriate blocking and tackling techniques is likely the single most important intervention in preventing recurrent burner syndrome or more serious cervical spine injuries.

## CERVICAL SPRAINS AND STRAINS

Simple stable cervical sprains and strains occur frequently in contact sports. Cervical strains that involve muscles and tendons, and cervical sprains that involve ligaments, occur as a result of rapid acceleration-deceleration or direct contact.

The athlete will complain of neck pain. The exam reveals tenderness generally along the cervical paraspinous muscles and the trapezius muscles. Cervical range of motion is compromised secondary to pain and muscle spasms. The neurologic exam evaluating strength, sensation, and reflexes of the upper extremities is normal.

Treatment is symptomatic with local application of ice, use of nonsteroidal antiinflammatory drugs, and modalities as indicated. Although it allows considerable motion, a soft cervical collar can provide symptomatic relief. Range of motion and strengthening exercises are added as tolerated. Return to play is allowed when the patient has pain-free cervical full range of motion and strength. It typically takes 3 to 7 days for the injury to resolve. A more prolonged duration or any change in symptoms suggests a need for further evaluation.

## ACUTE CERVICAL DISK HERNIATION

Fortunately, acute cervical disk herniation is rare in sports. When it occurs it typically results from axial loading of the cervical spine with resultant expression of disk fragments into the vertebral canal and/or foramen. This causes compromise of either the spinal cord or its nerve roots. It can be associated with a vertebral fracture or dislocation.

Regardless of the location of herniation, limitation of cervical range of motion is present. Movement, especially hyperextension of the neck, aggravates the pain. If the herniated disk encroaches on a nerve root, then motor weakness, sensory disturbances, and decreased reflexes corresponding to the specific level of herniation are seen. Central disk herniations may show involvement of bilateral upper extremities and/or the lower extremities. In the case of C3 and C4 acute disk herniations, transient quadriplegia may be the presenting sign. An acute anterior cervical cord injury syndrome has also been described. This presents as quadriplegia with loss of pain, temperature, and sensation. Vibratory, motion, and position sensations are preserved. These injuries should be treated as severe cervical injuries, with appropriate stabilization and transport procedures followed.

Chronic cervical intervertebral disk injury is thought to be commonplace in sports. This typically results in disk space narrowing or early degenerative changes. Range of motion and pain should determine playing status in these individuals.

## CERVICAL SPINAL CORD NEURAPRAXIA

Transient paraplegia or quadriplegia can occur without associated intervertebral disk herniation. It can be seen following forced hyperextension, hyperflexion, or axial loading.

Following the injury, immediate onset of motor paresis involving both arms, both legs, or all four extremities occurs. This is demonstrated as gross weakness or total paralysis. Associated sensory changes are exemplified by burning, tingling, and loss of sensation in the affected extremities. The symptoms are always bilateral. Neck pain is not present.

The episode is transient, with full recovery expected in minutes. Rare cases have required 36 to 48 hours, with full recovery following. The most consistent finding on radiographic evaluation is cervical spinal stenosis.

By itself, developmental cervical stenosis, with or without an associated episode of transient quadriplegia, is not an absolute contraindication to play. Return to play is considered once full cervical range of motion and full strength have returned with no neurologic abnormalities noted. A Cowboy collar, continued neck strengthening, and a reminder of the dangers of spearing are recommended. It is important that all parties concerned be aware of the inherent dangers of contact sports and that recommendations are based on currently available data.

There are compromising factors that emphasize the need for more conservative measures. Any associated signs of ligamentous instability, disk disease, congenital cervical anomalies, or spondylitic changes suggest a more serious problem. Also, MRI evidence of cord swelling or cord defect increases the risk for permanent damage. An athlete who has had more than one episode of transient quadriplegia or an episode that lasts more than 36 hours is placed in the increased risk group, with continuation in contact sports prohibited.

There is an additional entity referred to as spear tackler's spine that leads to disqualification from contact play. This term refers to a constellation of radiographic findings that include developmental cervical stenosis, persistent loss of lordosis, and spondylitic changes. The radiographic findings listed and the documentation of spear tackling techniques used are enough to prohibit one from participating in contact sports.

## LIGAMENTOUS INSTABILITY

Typically, cervical ligamentous instability involves the posterior soft tissue support system of the cervical spine. Axial compression or extreme flexion leads to disruption of the posterior ligaments. This can result in translation or angulation of the vertebral body with resultant compromise of the neural elements.

This injury may initially appear insignificant. Pain with cervical motion and associated muscle spasm are typical. Radiation of pain or symptoms into the trapezius or upper extremities may not be present acutely. The initial neurologic exam is often normal. Understandably, posterior ligament instability is often mistaken for a cervical sprain.

Routine cervical spine films including AP, lateral, and oblique views can be normal. It is important to remember that vertebral body fractures or dislocations are not required for an injury to be unstable. It may require cervical flexion and extension views to demonstrate the translation or angulation of the vertebral body that is causing the symptoms. Further studies including MRI are often required. Referral to a neurosurgeon or orthopedic spine surgeon is recommended.

## CERVICAL DISLOCATION

Cervical dislocations occur as a result of severe flexion and rotational forces. They may be unilateral or bilateral facet dislocations. With a unilateral facet dislocation, a rotational force significant enough to tear the facet joint capsule is required. If compression of a nerve root is involved, motor weakness and sensory loss in the so innervated muscle group is noted. A defect (step-off) may be noted on palpation of the cervical spine. These injuries are typically stable. Bilateral facet dislocations are obviously more severe injuries. Unlike a unilateral facet dislocation that requires extreme rotational forces, bilateral facet dislocations result from extreme flexion forces. This leads to disruption of intravertebral disks, posterior longitudinal ligaments, and the capsule of the associated facet joints. This is an unstable injury with associated neurologic deficits. Complete quadriplegia or sudden death can occur. These do require reduction and most often fusion. Cervical dislocations may occur in association with cervical fractures.

## CERVICAL SPINE FRACTURES

Cervical spine fractures along with cervical dislocations are associated with the highest mortality rate of all neck injuries. For ease of discussion, these are divided into upper (C1 to C2), mid (C3 to C4), and lower (C4 to C7) cervical spine injures.

Upper cervical spine fractures rarely occur in sports. Those that are considerations are briefly mentioned. A Jefferson's fracture is a burst fracture of the anterior and posterior arch of C1. This results from the crushing of the atlas (C1) by the occipital condyle as a result of axial loading forces. One third of these fractures are associated with C2 fractures. A hangman's fracture involves the posterior arch of the axis (C2). This potentially unstable fracture results from extension and distraction, or extension and axial loading, of the cervical spine. Fractures of the odontoid process also occur. The initial neurologic exam may be normal. Cervical tenderness is present and paraspinous muscle spasms are often palpable. Attempts at nodding or neck rotation are painful and resisted by the athlete. Any suspected upper cervical injury should be treated as potentially unstable and life threatening since the reticular activating system that controls respiration is located in this area.

Fractures involving the mid cervical (C3 to C4) vertebrae are rare. Disk herniations are more likely in this area than are fractures.

The lower cervical spine (C5 to C7) is the most common location for cervical fractures that occur in sports. These are typically compression fractures resulting from axial loading. There are five classifications, with type I (vertebral endplate fractures) and type II (anterior and inferior vertebral body fractures or teardrop lesions) considered stable. These have little potential for associated neural damage. Types III to V are more severe, with a substantial risk of neural damage leading to paralysis or sudden death. Any cervical spine tenderness or pain on attempted neck motion should be considered an unstable injury. Neurologic deficits are not necessarily present. The attempt is to prevent seemingly benign cervical injuries from becoming unstable cervical disasters.

## THE UNSTABLE CERVICAL SPINE

The unstable cervical spine is the most feared of all injuries in sports. It should be suspected in all injuries involving the head, neck, and upper trunk. Careful assessment and appropriate transport can help prevent a stable injury from becoming an unstable disaster.

An unconscious player or a player suspected of having a spine injury should receive the same initial management. A well-established plan with an educated training staff and coaching staff is essential. All should understand the importance of appropriate on-site management in the prevention of catastrophic injury. The team physician or athletic trainer should be designated as supervisor over the proceedings. It is ideal for each team member to know the basics:

- CPR
- Log roll technique
- Face mask removal
- Location of emergency equipment
- Method of notifying emergency support staff
- Appropriate lifting and carrying techniques

Necessary equipment should be readily available:

- Bolt cutters or sharp knife or scalpel
- Spine board

- Rigid cervical collar
- Oxygen
- Telephone

In the event that the injury is severe, knowledge regarding quick access to back-up support is essential:

- Ambulance or rescue squad
- Hospital equipped with appropriate radiologic facility
- Neurosurgeon or orthopedic spine surgeon

When a player goes down on the field with a suspected spine injury, a systematic evaluation of the athlete is crucial. Initially, an assessment for a patent airway, spontaneous breathing, and adequate circulation is carried out. If a deficit is noted, correction of the problem must be addressed first and foremost. This may require moving the athlete, which generally would not be recommended until further neurologic assessment.

To move an athlete with a suspected cervical spine injury, the log roll technique is recommended. This requires four people. The predesignated supervisor is responsible for stabilizing the head and neck and orchestrating the movement of the athlete. Other care givers are placed at the shoulders, hips, and knees. Manual stabilization of the neck is achieved by grasping the trapezius, clavicle, and scapula with the hands while supporting the head between the forearms. Once the head and neck are stabilized and the supervisor gives the go-ahead, the athlete is rolled toward the care givers while maintaining body alignment. Ideally the athlete is rolled directly on a spine board.

Once in the supine position, stabilization of the athlete's head and neck is maintained. A reassessment of airway and breathing is made. If CPR is indicated, the face mask is removed using bolt cutters for the older model helmets and a sharp knife or scalpel for the newer helmets that have plastic loop attachments for the face masks. Do not remove the helmet or the chin straps at this time. Once the face mask is removed, rescue breathing is initiated using the jaw thrust maneuver to open the airway. This maneuver is performed by the supervisor, who grasps the angle of the lower jaw and lifts with both hands, thus displacing the mandible upward with only minimal extension of the neck. CPR is continued until a transport crew has arrived.

Once a transport crew has arrived the athlete, if not previously placed on a spine board, should be placed on one, again using the log roll technique. The board is then lifted by four individuals, one at each corner of the spine board. The team supervisor maintains head and neck stability and provides the directive on when to move.

Transport to a facility with necessary radiographic capabilities and appropriate neurosurgical or orthopedic spine consultation is crucial. A crude neurologic assessment using the Glasgow Coma Scale is appropriate before transport. Delay in order to perform a more thorough neurologic exam is not warranted.

Once in an appropriate medical facility and after the institution of more permanent immobilization techniques, the chin strap and helmet can be removed. This requires two individuals, one supporting the cervical spine and the other spreading the helmet from the sides and removing it in a straight line from the spine. Definitive x-rays are then performed to rule out fractures or instability. A comprehensive neurologic exam follows. In those individuals with neurologic deficits noted or in those athletes who are regarded with a high index of suspicion for cord trauma, intravenous steroids are recommended. Methylprednisolone given as an intravenous bolus of 30 mg/kg over a 15-minute period is advised. This is followed by a continuous infusion of 5.4 mg/kg/hr for a period of 24 hours. Studies have shown that significant improvement in neurologic recovery has been noted in individuals with traumatic cord injuries who receive this medication within the initial 8-hour period. Neurosurgical or orthopedic spine consultation should be available.

For the athlete who goes down but is conscious, with no signs of cardiorespiratory problems, a quick neurologic assessment on the field is appropriate. The athlete should not be moved until this is completed. The athlete should be asked basic questions concerning the mechanism of injury and quality and location of pain:

- Was he or she knocked unconscious?
- Is there pain in the neck?
- Is there pain in any extremity?
- Is there numbness or tingling in any extremity?
- Can he or she move all extremities?

A cursory exam follows:

- Palpation of the cervical spine
- Assessment of movement in all extremities
- Assessment of sensation in all extremities

If the athlete's responses to questioning or the physician's findings upon completion of the cursory exam are all normal, then the athlete may walk with assistance to the sideline for a more complete neurologic assessment. If, however, there are any abnormal responses or findings, then transport and further evaluation, as for an unstable spine, is recommended.

The athlete whose on-field assessment allows him or her to walk to the sideline requires a complete cervical spine and neurologic evaluation. Any significant neurologic deficit, or cervical spine pain or tenderness to palpation, is treated as an unstable spine and transported accordingly. There are certain red flags that should alert one to a possible unstable cervical spine:

- Tender or painful cervical spine
- Palpable defect of the cervical spine
- Loss of motion of the cervical spine
- Prolonged burner syndrome
- Bilateral burner syndrome
- Any involvement of the lower extremities

If any of these signs or symptoms are present the player should not be allowed to play. A more complete neurologic evaluation with appropriate radiographic studies, and possibly neurologic consultation, is recommended.

It is important to keep in mind that when treating an athlete with a suspected cervical spine injury, a well-thought-out plan can prevent a seemingly minor injury from becoming a disaster. A well-organized staff with appropriate equipment is essential. The physician or athletic trainer who is responsible for the initial assessment should remain calm and not be rushed by the fury of the game. If evaluation suggests a possible cervical spine injury, then return to play should not be allowed. The adage "When in doubt, keep them out" rings especially true for neck injuries.

## Bibliography

Birrer RB: After a blow to the head, *Emerg Med Clin North Am* 23:56-66, 1991.

Bruno LA, Gennarelli TA, Torg JS: Head injuries. In Torg JS, Welsh RP, Shepard RJ, editors: *Current therapies in sports medicine*, ed 2, Toronto, 1990, BC Decker.

Cantu RC: A randomized, controlled trial of methylprednisolone or naloxone in the treatment of acute spinal-cord injury, *New Engl J Med* 322:1405-1411, 1990.

Cantu RC: Criteria for return to competition after a closed head injury. In Torg JS, editor: *Athletic injuries to the head, neck, and face*, ed 2, St Louis, 1991, Mosby–Year Book.

Jane JA, Rimel RW, Pobereskin LH et al: Outcome and pathology of head injury. In Grossman RG, Gilden PL, editors: *Head injury: basic and clinical aspects*, New York, 1982, Raven Press.

Reid DC, editor: *Sports injury assessment and rehabilitation*, New York, 1992, Churchill Livingstone.

Salcman M, Geisler FH: Emergency: head trauma, *Hosp Med* 29:78-111, 1993.

Vegso JJ, Lehman RC: Field evaluation and management of head and neck injuries, *Clin Sports Med* 6:1-15, 1987.

# Chapter 2

# Ocular and periocular trauma

Ferenc Kuhn
C. Douglas Witherspoon
Robert Morris
Gregg Kaiser

Overall, the visual system provides about two thirds of the sensory information reaching us from the outside world. For certain activities, such as athletic competition, this proportion is even higher. Optimum functioning of each eye and an effective cooperation between the two eyes (binocular stereoscopic vision) are necessary in most sports for the athlete to perform to the maximum potential. If a part of the peripheral visual field is lost (e.g., following retinal detachment or traumatic retinopathy) or the central vision is severely diminished (e.g., as a result of traumatic macular hole or contusion maculopathy), not only can such an event end a career in a particular sport, but there may be tragic consequences for the individual's entire life.

Prevention of eye injuries through education, training, protective rules and regulations, and appropriate physical measures (e.g., safety eyewear) is more effective and less expensive (with respect to direct costs, disabled time, and so on) than treatment after the fact. Such preventive activities are therefore in the best interest of the player. Should preventive measures fail, proper and timely treatment of eye injuries is critical to keep disability at a minimum and return a player to optimum performance as soon as possible.

The eye is well protected in the bony orbit. Paradoxically, however, the globe must turn toward the potential source of harm to fulfill its desired function, and thus it becomes highly vulnerable to injury. This vulnerability is particularly true in sport activities where the very object of regard (e.g., a ball or an opposing player) is usually the agent of injury. This chapter provides some basic guidelines for on-field evaluation of the player with a suspected eye injury and makes recommendations about first aid, the need for further treatment, if any, and the athlete's ability to return to play.

## MECHANISM OF INJURY

There are several factors that determine whether a potentially injurious agent, under a certain set of circumstances, will leave an eye unharmed or inflict physical injury. These factors include the shape, mass, and speed of the agent; the site of impact; the efficacy of the defensive reflexes (e.g., squeezing the eyelids); the protective equipment; and the condition of the globe (e.g., whether it has experienced previous trauma or surgery, or whether high myopia is present). The same agent, acting in different situations under nearly identical circumstances, may cause damage to one eye and leave another unharmed.

An object causes a contusion injury when tissue damage occurs without the creation of a full-thickness disruption of the eyewall (i.e., the cornea and the sclera; see Fig. 2-1). Consequently, severe intraocular damage may be present in an eye with a normal external appearance. Contusion injuries usually are caused by blunt objects (e.g., a tennis ball or another player's arm) that have their energy spread over a relatively large contact area. Partial thickness globe injuries usually are caused by sharp objects that have relatively less momentum and/or contact the eye

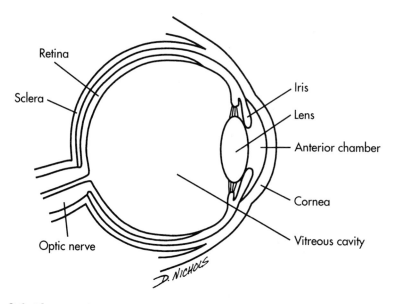

**Fig. 2-1.** The most important tissues of the eyeball. The wall is made up of the cornea and the sclera. Most of the sclera is lined on the inside by the choroid and the retina. The anterior chamber is bordered by the cornea, the iris, and the lens. The space between the iris, the lens, and the retina is called the vitreous cavity and is normally completely occupied by the vitreous gel.

at an angle (e.g., a tangential path of contact with another player's fingernail). The object splits open the cornea—or, less frequently, the sclera—to a limited depth.

An object with substantial momentum often creates an open globe injury. If the object is blunt the impact force may dramatically elevate the intraocular pressure. The eye eventually gives way at its weakest point, which is not necessarily at the site of the impact. The resulting rupture often is the most severe type of injury since it is usually associated with significant loss of intraocular contents—uvea, vitreous, retina, and so on. A typical example of a blunt object that can cause such an injury is a racquetball, which is small enough to fit into the orbital aperture to allow the transmission of most of its kinetic energy to the globe.

A sharp object, on the other hand, usually lacerates the cornea and/or the sclera at the impact site. The sharp object either entirely penetrates the eyewall without actually being retained intraocularly (e.g., a spike from a running shoe) or is physically retained within the globe and becomes an intraocular foreign body (e.g., a ricocheted fragment of a BB gun pellet). Finally, the energy of the object may be so great (e.g., the force of a shotgun pellet) that it completely traverses the eye, creating a perforating injury. Figure 2-2 provides an overview of these major categories of eye injury.

In addition to injuries to the globe itself, the eyelids may become lacerated, with or without involvement of the tear ducts; the bony orbit may

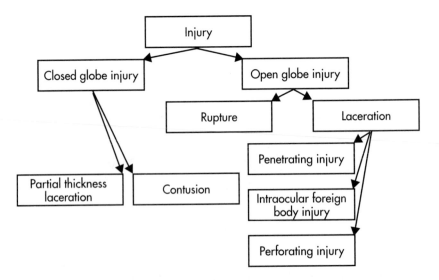

**Fig. 2-2.** Injury types involving the eyeball.

be fractured; the extraocular muscles may become damaged; and the optic nerve may sustain direct or indirect injuries.

## CLINICAL DIAGNOSIS

### SUBJECTIVE

The list of symptoms signaling significant eye and/or adnexal injury is rather limited:

1. *Eyelid swelling*: hemorrhage; edema
2. *Ptosis*: eyelid swelling; nerve lesion
3. *Foreign body sensation; tearing; or less frequently, burning*: presence of a surface foreign body either on the bulbar conjunctiva or on the conjunctiva lining the inner surface of the eyelids; corneal abrasion-erosion
4. *Pain*: wound of the eyelid, conjunctiva, or cornea; direct trauma involving the uveal tissue; increased intraocular or intraorbital pressure
5. *Mobile spots*: posterior vitreous detachment; vitreous hemorrhage; retinal break with operculum
6. *Flashes of light*: mechanical trauma; retinal break; retinal detachment
7. *Double vision*: acute imbalance of extraocular muscle(s); orbital fracture; orbital hemorrhage; lens dislocation
8. *Loss of visual field*: narrowed eyelid fissure (eyelid swelling, ptosis; see above); corneal opacity; traumatic cataract; vitreous hemorrhage; retinal hemorrhage; retinal detachment
9. *Blurred-decreased-lost vision*: corneal opacity; hyphema; mydriasis; lens dislocation; traumatic cataract; vitreous hemorrhage; macular edema; macular hemorrhage; retinal detachment involving the macula; optic nerve compression; optic nerve avulsion

Pain involving the eye or periocular structures and decreased visual acuity (central vision) are the most common complaints and may be seen in a large variety of pathologic conditions. Injured patients also frequently complain of loss of peripheral vision and/or of double vision (diplopia). Another common symptom is sensitivity to light (photophobia). This may be associated with foreign body sensation, tearing, or burning in or around the globe. An increased degree of floaters or flashing lights (photopsia) may signal the onset of severe retinal damage such as a retinal tear or detachment.

### OBJECTIVE

Many kinds of eye injuries are easily detected in an ocular examination that do not require the use of specialized equipment. The eyelids may be swollen or bruised. Droopiness of the eyelid could signal damage to the extraocular muscles or neurologic injury. Excessive tearing may be caused by irritation secondary to any major ocular injury, but damage to the lacrimal drainage system should be suspected if the injury involves the medial canthal region. Other external signs of ocular injury include swelling, bleeding, or bruising of the eye or periocular structures; abnormal positioning of the globe (e.g., enophthalmos, exophthalmos); absence of normal, parallel eye movements; and abnormal discoloration of the sclera (usually red, blue, or black). Displaced facial fractures may be visible externally. Intraocular signs that are often visible with a penlight examination include blood within the anterior chamber of the eye (hyphema), flattening of the anterior chamber or obvious disorganization of the globe, abnormal pupillary reaction, and unequal or irregular pupils.

Listed here are only those signs that do not require special equipment (slit lamp, ophthalmoscope, and so on) to be detected:

1. *Eyelid swelling*: hemorrhage; edema
2. *Ptosis*: eyelid swelling; nerve lesion
3. *Excessive tearing*: severed (inferior) tear duct
4. *Bleeding*: lid laceration; conjunctival wound; open globe injury with severe intraocular hemorrhage
5. *Dispositioned globe*: acute imbalance of extraocular muscles; orbital fracture; orbital hemorrhage
6. *"Red eye"*: subconjunctival hemorrhage; conjunctival injection usually as a result of mechanical trauma; corneal-conjunctival foreign body
7. *Circumscribed blue discoloration of sclera*: open globe injury (uveal tissue visible)
8. *Shallow anterior chamber*: dislocated lens; intraocular hemorrhage
9. *Hyphema*: ruptured iris or ciliary vessels; less frequently, blood originates in the posterior segment
10. *Mydriasis and/or irregularly shaped pupil*: mechanical trauma to iris-nerve; dislocated lens
11. *Abnormal shape of, or shrunken, eye*: open globe injury with loss of intraocular globe contents

## DIFFERENTIAL DIAGNOSIS

A summary of the major signs and symptoms commonly seen in eye injuries and the differential diagnoses associated with each are listed in Table 4.

*Text continued on p. 25*

**Table 4**
**DIFFERENTIAL DIAGNOSES OF VARIOUS SIGNS AND SYMPTOMS OF OCULAR AND PERIOCULAR TRAUMA**

| Sign or symptom | Differential diagnosis |
|---|---|
| Foreign body sensation | Conjunctival-corneal foreign body<br>Corneal abrasion<br>Eyelash rubbing against cornea or conjunctiva<br>*Look for a foreign body on the cornea, conjunctival cul-de-sac, or inner surface of the everted upper eyelid; check for an eyelash that is turned inward.*<br>*Examine the cornea and conjunctiva with fluorescein dye, if possible.* |
| Tearing | Conjunctival-corneal foreign body<br>Corneal abrasion<br>Eyelash rubbing against cornea or conjunctiva<br>Mechanical-chemical trauma to the eye with or without causing wound(s)<br>*Look for a foreign body on the cornea, conjunctival cul-de-sac, or inner surface of the everted upper eyelid; check for an eyelash that is turned inward.* |
| Burning | Loss of corneal-conjunctival epithelium<br>*Conjunctival epithelial loss causes only a minor burning sensation and is difficult to visualize; corneal epithelial loss causes the distortion of an image reflected from the corneal surface.* |
| Pain | Loss of corneal epithelium (severe) or conjunctival epithelium (mild)<br>Visible wounds of globe or lids<br>Fracture of bony orbit<br>"Deep": intraocular or intraorbital pathology (e.g., hemorrhage)<br>Any serious open or closed globe injury causing tissue damage<br>*A cornea denuded of its epithelium causes extreme pain. The pain and the severity of an eye injury are not necessarily directly related.* |
| Photophobia (sensitivity to light) | Mydriasis (enlarged pupil)<br>Any wound of the eye<br>Corneal abrasion<br>Any severe blunt injury (traumatic uveitis)<br>*All are easily recognizable; the pupil may not constrict when exposed to light.* |

*Continued*

**Table 4—cont'd**
**DIFFERENTIAL DIAGNOSES OF VARIOUS SIGNS AND**
**SYMPTOMS OF OCULAR AND PERIOCULAR TRAUMA**

| Sign or symptom | Differential diagnosis |
| --- | --- |
| Mobile floating spots | *These are visible usually when looking at a white surface; they may be insignificant or very important and are impossible to determine without special equipment.* |
| Flashes of light (photopsia) | Mechanical trauma (hitting the eye) |
| | Retinal break |
| | Retinal detachment |
| | *If the cause is external trauma, the flashes are concurrent and do not return subsequently; if the cause is a retinal pathology, the flashes usually recur with sudden eye movements.* |
| Double vision | Extraocular muscle(s) damage or the nerve severed |
| | Orbital fracture |
| | Orbital hemorrhage |
| | Lens dislocation |
| | *If the eye's movement is restricted only in certain directions and double vision presents only in those directions, it is probably a muscle problem or is caused by an orbital (blow out) fracture. An orbital hemorrhage usually results in limited eye movement in all directions. If the lens is dislocated, the eye's movements are unrestricted.* |
| | *Double vision rarely is present monocularly; this is usually caused by a dislocated lens.* |
| Loss of visual field | Narrowed eyelid fissure |
| | Corneal opacity |
| | Traumatic cataract |
| | Vitreous hemorrhage |
| | Retinal hemorrhage |
| | Retinal detachment |
| | *Loss of visual field is obvious if the eyelids do not open sufficiently or if the cornea is opaque; a white reflex may indicate that a cataract is present although it is not a reliable sign. The other conditions require special equipment to differentiate.* |

**Table 4—cont'd**
## DIFFERENTIAL DIAGNOSES OF VARIOUS SIGNS AND SYMPTOMS OF OCULAR AND PERIOCULAR TRAUMA

| Sign or symptom | Differential diagnosis |
|---|---|
| Blurred, decreased, or complete absence of vision | See the diagnosis list on p. 22. *Blood in the anterior chamber usually is recognizable when the player is not in a horizontal position. The other conditions require special equipment to differentiate.* |
| Eyelid swelling | Hemorrhage<br>Edema<br>*It is very difficult to make a distinction acutely; with time, the hemorrhage usually causes lid discoloration. Both are insignificant by themselves but may indicate severe underlying conditions. If air is also present (crepitation), a sinus probably is fractured.* |
| Ptosis | Eyelid swelling<br>Nerve lesion<br>*If the lid is swollen, its weight gradually overcomes the elevator muscle's power, but some function is retained. A nerve lesion causes an all-or-nothing type of function loss.* |
| Excessive tearing | Severed (inferior) tear duct<br>*The innermost portion of the lid is torn, medial to the lacrimal punctum.* |
| Bleeding | Lid laceration<br>Conjunctival wound<br>Open globe injury with severe intraocular hemorrhage<br>*The cause of the hemorrhage may appear obvious, but one area can mask the other (e.g., a conjunctival bleeding making a scleral wound invisible).* |
| Dispositioned globe | Acute imbalance of extraocular muscles<br>Orbital fracture<br>Orbital hemorrhage<br>*Whereas a nonfunctioning muscle restricts the globe's mobility in certain direction(s), an orbital fracture literally "sinks" the eye by removing part of its support from underneath. A hemorrhage behind the globe usually pushes it straight forward (proptosis). Remember that the majority of maxillofacial fractures have associated eye injuries.* |

*Continued*

**Table 4—cont'd**
**DIFFERENTIAL DIAGNOSES OF VARIOUS SIGNS AND
SYMPTOMS OF OCULAR AND PERIOCULAR TRAUMA**

| Sign or symptom | Differential diagnosis |
|---|---|
| "Red eye" | Subconjunctival hemorrhage<br>Conjunctival injection (mechanical trauma)<br>Corneal-conjunctival foreign body<br>*A hemorrhage gives a more universal appearance of red. Irritation causes the individual blood vessels to dilate. One of the most frequent causes of irritation is a foreign body (additional symptoms are usually involved; see* Foreign body sensation, p. 21). |
| Circumscribed blue discoloration of sclera | Open globe injury with uveal prolapse<br>*Though foreign objects also may appear as a discoloration over the normally white sclera, prolapse of the uvea has a distinctive dark blue color; and the wound of the eyeball is usually also visible.* |
| Shallow anterior chamber | Dislocated lens<br>Intraocular hemorrhage<br>*The condition is easily recognizable: the iris is very close to the cornea. The cause is usually a dislocated lens, but the exact diagnosis may require special equipment.* |
| Hyphema | *Though hyphema usually is caused by closed globe injuries, presence of an open wound must be excluded.* |
| Mydriasis and/or irregularly shaped pupil | Mechanical trauma to iris and its nervous innervation<br>Dislocated lens<br>*If the lens is not seen "stuck" in the pupil, mechanical trauma to the iris or nerve is the cause (this is the case in the vast majority of the situations).* |
| Abnormal shape of, or shrunken, eye | *No condition other than an open globe injury with loss of intraocular globe contents gives this appearance.* |

The differential diagnosis of most conditions is made easier by comparing the player's two eyes; usually only one is involved in the injury. Should both eyes be affected, another individual should serve as the control.

## ON-FIELD ASSESSMENT, TREATMENT, AND RETURN-TO-PLAY CRITERIA

An initial on-field assessment is appropriate to evaluate a suspected eye injury and to screen for other injuries that may prevent safe movement of the athlete. A player who is suspected of having an eye injury should be evaluated thoroughly on the sideline with sufficient time allowed to determine if a significant eye injury is indeed present, and to administer first aid if indicated. Then a decision can be made as to whether the athlete can return to play or is in need of an in-depth evaluation by an eye trauma surgeon who is experienced in the management of sports-related eye injuries.

In general no player should be examined, much less treated, on the actual field. The player should be brought off the field, with intervention conducted along the sideline. This maneuver eliminates the game's pressure and reduces the possibility of missing an important diagnosis.

The examination begins with a careful, detailed, but specific history. The mechanism of injury should be determined. Symptoms should be elicited with special attention given to the key symptoms listed in Table 4. Note what happened, how the eye may have been injured, what the symptoms are and were, and any changes in the symptoms that may have occurred since the time of injury. The presence of any pain or visual symptoms must be questioned. Following the history the sideline physical examination is carried out to screen for any (significant) eye injury. The major signs and symptoms of eye injuries are fairly limited, so this examination can be performed in a short period of time with a high level of confidence that most significant eye injuries will be discovered.

The sideline examination often is difficult because of the natural protective mechanisms that most individuals possess with respect to their eyes. The player should be reassured that neither pain nor harm will be inflicted during the examination. The player also should be reassured of the importance of a good examination. It is critical to remember that there is an increased risk of extrusion of intraocular contents if pressure is placed inadvertently on the globe either by the injured player squeezing the eyelids or by the person conducting the examination. If the player is not counseled properly ("Keep both of your eyes open so that I can easily see what's wrong; don't squeeze"), the original injury can be compounded. The natural reflex is to squeeze the lids tight when threatened. In the presence of an open globe injury, squeezing can lead to the loss of intraocular contents, which may result in potentially tragic consequences. If the player's problem is obvious (e.g., a conjunctival foreign body), there is no need to perform a complete examination. Any abnormality found in assessing these basic criteria should make the examiner suspect that significant eye injury exists.

If an obvious and serious abnormality is discovered, triage the player to an eye trauma specialist. Keep in mind, though, that multiple eye injuries may be present. A complete on-field eye screening examination is described here.

Optimally the eye and adnexa are first examined without physical contact. The lids are inspected for shape, symmetry, swelling, discoloration, and wounds. Next the periocular area and tissues, including the facial bones, are observed and palpated for a step sign or any asymmetry that may indicate an orbital fracture. The globe's position is then compared with the contralateral globe for any sign of displacement. If none is noted, the globe's overall position is confirmed.

Then the surface of the globe is checked for signs of injury. Staining with fluorescein dye often is the only effective way of demonstrating a corneal abrasion, which is one of the most common sports-related eye injuries. An estimate of the visual acuity can be obtained by using a near vision screening card; any small-print text; or small, distant objects that are clearly visible to the examiner. The peripheral visual field may be checked by having the examiner face the player eye-to-eye (i.e., left eye of the player aligns with the right eye of the examiner). The examiner moves a hand, midway from the player, from the outside inward until seen by the player. Both the player and the examiner should notice the moving hand simultaneously. The athlete's eyes should be directed toward all fields of gaze to check for normal mobility. Additionally, the player should be instructed to report any symptoms of double vision that were precipitated by these fields of gaze. The pupil's reaction to light may be checked with a penlight or by simply covering and uncovering the eye under bright illumination. The pupils should be equal in size, should be round in shape, and should respond (i.e., constrict) briskly to light.

If the globe is not obviously open, but an occult wound cannot be excluded confidently, an experienced examiner may carefully check the intraocular pressure. In all cases care should be taken to avoid excessive pressure on the globe if an open globe injury cannot be excluded. If the examiner is uncertain about the degree of injury to the globe, then consultation with a more experienced examiner should be obtained to prevent making the situation worse.

Table 5 provides an overview of the specific actions that should be taken in the most common types of eye injury cases. A few general precautions, however, always must be kept in mind when evaluating a player on the sideline:

- No eye should be examined with dirty hands. For the protection of both the injured player and the examiner, sterile examination gloves should be used if at all possible.

**Table 5**
**ON-FIELD (SIDELINE) MANAGEMENT OF THE MOST**
**COMMON EYE INJURIES**

| Injury | Management |
|---|---|
| Eyelid wound | Use moist gauze. |
| | Apply cold compress. |
| | NO RETURN TO PLAY unless the wound is very small and does not involve the lid margins. The wound can then be disinfected and temporarily taped over. |
| | *Refer the athlete to an eye trauma surgeon.* |
| Conjunctival abrasion | Apply topical antibiotics if the abrasion is severe. |
| | A patch is rarely necessary. |
| | RETURN TO PLAY. |
| Corneal abrasion | Apply topical antibiotics and cycloplegics if the abrasion is severe. |
| | Do not use topical analgesics. |
| | Use a patch if the pain or tearing is severe. |
| | RETURN TO PLAY if the pain is not too severe. |
| | *Refer the athlete to an ophthalmologist if symptoms persist and inflammation ensues.* |
| Superficial corneal foreign body | Irrigate it off. |
| | If unsuccessful (use topical analgetics if necessary) carefully remove the foreign body using a clean cloth or sterile cotton-tipped applicator. |
| | Apply topical antibiotics. |
| | Use a patch if a large area of corneal abrasion is present. |
| | RETURN TO PLAY if the pain is not too severe. |
| | *Refer the athlete to an ophthalmologist if the symptoms persist and inflammation ensues.* |
| Superficial conjunctival foreign body | Irrigate it. |
| | If unsuccessful (use topical analgetics if necessary), carefully remove the foreign body using a clean cloth or sterile cotton-tipped applicator; the upper lid may have to be pulled down and forward or everted. |
| | Topical antibiotics and patching are rarely necessary (only if a large area of corneal abrasion is present). |
| | RETURN TO PLAY if the pain is not too severe. |

*Continued*

**Table 5—cont'd**
**ON-FIELD (SIDELINE) MANAGEMENT OF THE MOST**
**COMMON EYE INJURIES**

| Injury | Management |
|---|---|
| Subconjunctival hemorrhage | No treatment is necessary if no other injury is present. RETURN TO PLAY. |
| Orbital fracture | Patch. NO RETURN TO PLAY. *Refer the athlete to an eye trauma surgeon.* |
| Orbital hemorrhage | NO RETURN TO PLAY. *Refer the athlete to an eye trauma surgeon. If severe pain and gradual loss of vision are present, treat the injury as an emergency.* |
| Optic nerve injury | NO RETURN TO PLAY. *Refer the athlete to an eye trauma surgeon.* |
| Closed globe injuries | *Consider using a protective patch or shield.* |
| *Partial thickness corneal-scleral laceration* | NO RETURN TO PLAY. *Refer the athlete to an eye trauma surgeon.* |
| *Hyphema* | |
| *Iris rupture or dialysis* | |
| *Cyclodialysis cleft* | |
| *Angle recession or glaucoma* | |
| *Traumatic cataract* | |
| *Dislocated lens* | |
| *Vitreous hemorrhage* | |
| *Contusion retinopathy or macular hole* | |
| *Retinal break or detachment* | |
| Open globe injuries | Use a protective patch or shield. |
| *Corneal-scleral rupture or laceration* | Control the pain, anxiety, and nausea; if possible, do not use oral medications. |
| *Intraocular foreign body* | Do not extract a protruding foreign body. |
| *Any of the tissue lesions listed under* Closed globe injuries, *above* | Provide counseling. NO RETURN TO PLAY. *Immediately refer the athlete to an eye trauma surgeon.* |

- No existing condition should be made more severe by trying to get an accurate diagnosis (e.g., if the globe is open there is no need to determine how posteriorly the scleral wound extends).
- If an injury is indeed present, always remember that it is not simply a tissue-organ that is damaged, but rather a complete individual. Additional injuries may be present. Typically, patients with eye injuries are anxious and concerned about their athletic career and potential disability. If the player's general condition is not controlled and properly managed (pain, nausea, and so on), a dramatic worsening of the injury can result through elevation of the intraocular pressure. If possible, intramuscular or intravenous injections, rather than pills, should be used to minimize the pain and eliminate vomiting.
- It is safer, from a medical and a legal standpoint, to err on the "too cautious" side. Presuming an injury to be more severe than it really is may result in failure to return the player to the field during a particular game. However, failure to recognize the true severity of the condition and prematurely returning the player to the field may result in the loss of an eye and may deny the player the ability to compete in the future.

## CONCLUSION

Though the past two decades have seen a dramatic increase in the salvage rate of even the most severely injured eyes, it remains impossible to save all traumatized globes. Furthermore, even less severe injuries may result in permanent, partial visual disabilities. Additionally, there is often significant psychological distress associated with sight-threatening injuries that may prematurely end an athlete's career and cause significant disability in general. Therefore it is highly preferable to prevent these injuries through the use of appropriate prevention strategies. Even if preventive devices at first appear to interfere with performance, careful consideration is in order. Prejudice may play a more important role in declining safety eyewear than the presumed handicap. If the goalie in ice hockey can see a fast-traveling puck despite the face mask, surely a basketball player should not feel visually hindered by wearing polycarbonate goggles to protect something of which even the best player has only two—eyeballs.

# Chapter 3

# Exercise-induced allergic reactions

Mark Hutchens

Allergy is a hypersensitive state resulting from exposure to specific allergens. Sports and exercise may place an individual at risk for increased exposure to specific allergens and may cause significant symptoms. These symptoms may result from exposure to airborne allergens or from contact with specific sport equipment and include allergic conjunctivitis, allergic rhinitis, and atopic dermatitis. These symptoms can become severe enough to affect performance. Treatment options include avoidance techniques, desensitization, and pharmacotherapy. (See the box on p. 31.) Antihistamines and topical corticosteroids are very effective in controlling most symptoms. Sympathomimetic amines are banned by the International Olympic Committee (IOC) and should be avoided in athletes competing internationally. Likewise, international athletes should be warned that these substances are commonly used in over-the-counter medications.

In addition to developing the common allergy symptoms listed above, athletes are also at risk for developing symptoms as a result of their exercise. It is well recognized that exercise can be a stimulus for allergic reactions such as exercise-induced bronchospasm, urticaria, and anaphylaxis. The remainder of this chapter discusses the recognition and management of these exercise-induced allergic reactions.

## EXERCISE-INDUCED BRONCHOSPASM

Exercise-induced bronchospasm (EIB), also known as exercise-induced asthma (EIA), is characterized by a transient airflow obstruction following several minutes of strenuous exercise. EIB is a common clinical entity that may be responsible for exercise intolerance in many people. It occurs in 80% to 90% of known asthmatics, but it also occurs in 12% to 15% of the general population. Individuals with other atopic symptoms are at

## COMMON MEDICATIONS USED FOR ALLERGIC REACTIONS

**Antihistamines**
Astemizole (Hismanal)
Chlorpheniramine maleate
Clemastine (Tavist)
Diphenhydramine (Benadryl)
Terfenadine (Seldane)
**Decongestants**
Ephedrine*
Phenylephrine*
Phenylpropanolamine*
Pseudoephedrine*
**Inhaled β-Agonists**
Albuterol (Proventil, Ventolin)†
Terbutaline (Brethaire)†
Salmeterol (Serevent)†
Metaproterenol (Alupent, Metaprel)*
Pirbuterol (Maxair)*
**Cromolyn sodium (Intal, Nasalcrom)**
**Ipratropium bromide (Atrovent)**
**Inhaled corticosteroids†**
Beclomethasone (Beclovent, Beconase, Vanceril, Vancenase)
Flunisolide (Aerobid, Nasalide)
Triamcinolone (Azmacort)

*Banned by the IOC. Contact the United States Olympic Committe (USOC) for a complete list of banned substances.
†Requires that written notification from the prescribing physician be sent before competing in IOC-USOC events.

high risk for EIB, with 35% to 40% of that population being affected. Approximately 10% of athletes have EIB.

Obvious symptoms of EIB are wheezing, shortness of breath, and chest tightness after strenuous exercise. More subtle symptoms include a decrease in exercise tolerance, mild chest discomfort, frequent upper respiratory infection (URI) symptoms, and decreased energy. There is often a refractory period in which there is less bronchospasm with repeated exercise within 2 hours after the initial episode. Some may experience a late phase response following recovery. This may occur 4 to 12 hours after exercise and generally disappears within 24 hours.

The diagnosis of EIB is made by performing an exercise challenge test. The individual must exercise for 5 to 8 minutes at an intensity sufficient to raise the heart rate to 80% to 90% of the predicted maximum. A diagnosis of EIB is made if there is a 10% or greater reduction in forced expiratory volume in 1 second ($FEV_1$) or peak expiratory flow rate (PEFR). Using standard methodologic guidelines, the exercise challenge test can be performed in a laboratory on a treadmill or bicycle ergometer; but the test may be more sensitive with free-running in the environment where the athlete is most often exposed.

There is a greater risk of EIB in individuals with a personal or family history of asthma or other atopic symptoms. Bronchospasm is more easily provoked by such environmental conditions as low humidity, cold air, and allergen- or chemically polluted air. Sports that require continuous exertion at high aerobic capacity in the above-mentioned conditions present the greatest risk for provoking EIB.

The exact pathophysiology of EIB is unknown. Several theories exist:
1. Exercise-induced release of mediators from mast cells and granulocytes
2. Sympathetic mediation through vagus nerve stimulation
3. Respiratory heat loss
4. Respiratory water loss

The correct theory may be a combination of these. As vigorous exercise increases ventilatory rate there is a loss of respiratory heat and water. This in turn stimulates a cholinergic response and release of chemical mediators that cause bronchospasm. Although the exact mechanism is yet to be proven, it is clear that certain individuals are predisposed to bronchospasm with exercise in certain environmental conditions.

Nonpharmacologic treatment of EIB involves avoidance of exercise in a cold, dry environment or in polluted air. A face mask can often be used to filter air pollutants and to warm inspired air. Choice of sport may also influence the severity of EIB, with indoor swimming being the least provocative aerobic exercise. Good baseline aerobic conditioning seems to decrease the severity of the disease. An adequate warm-up period before exercising will decrease the amount of bronchospasm. (See the box on p. 33.)

Often, nonpharmacologic treatment is not sufficient or is impractical, and medication is needed to control bronchospasm. The drug of choice for EIB is an inhaled ß-agonist (albuterol, terbutaline, metaproterenol, pirbuterol). These drugs may be used for prophylaxis before exercise or as rescue therapy for acute bronchospasm. Typically they are used 20 to 30 minutes before exercise to prevent bronchospasm. Inhaled cromolyn sodium may also be used before exercise but is generally less effective than the ß-agonists. Both agents may be used together in refractory

## PRECOMPETITION PROPHYLAXIS OF EXERCISE-INDUCED BRONCHOSPASM

Premedicate 45 to 60 minutes before the competition with an inhaled ß-agonist and/or cromolyn sodium.

Start the warm-up with 10 to 15 minutes of gentle stretching.

Perform 5 to 10 minutes of aerobic exercise (easy jog) to raise the heart rate to 50% to 60% of the predicted maximum.

Perform a cool-down.

Administer an inhaled ß-agonist and/or cromolyn sodium 15 to 20 minutes before the competition.

patients and may work synergistically to control bronchospasm. Inhaled anticholinergic agents such as ipratropium bromide may be effective in EIB but must be used 1 hour before exercise. Sustained-release theophylline agents may have some benefit. Inhaled corticosteroids are not effective in controlling acute bronchospasm resulting from exercise, but they may be needed in some individuals as maintenance therapy when symptoms are not controlled with preexercise medication. Other agents that may be effective in controlling bronchospasm include newer generation antihistamines (terfenadine, astemizole) and calcium channel blockers.

Rules and regulations of the IOC must be adhered to when treating athletes competing in IOC-USOC events. As of January 1997, three ß-agonists are permitted by inhalation, but only with written notification from the prescribing physician sent before the competition. These three ß-agonists are albuterol, terbutaline, and salmeterol. All other ß-agonists are banned. Inhaled corticosteroids also require that written notification be sent before the competition. Oral, rectal, intramuscular, and intravenous corticosteroids are banned. Over-the-counter medications for asthma should be avoided since many contain banned substances such as sympathomimetic amines.

## EXERCISE-INDUCED URTICARIA

Exercise-induced urticaria (EIU) is characterized by the development of small (< 5 mm) pruritic papular wheals during or following exercise. Wheals generally first occur on the trunk and neck and then spread to the entire body. EIU is not associated with systemic reactions such as wheezing, gastrointestinal symptoms, or vascular collapse; and EIU is usually self-limiting. These lesions may also be induced by heat, fever, hot showers, and anxiety.

The mechanism of EIU is unknown. Some researchers have shown an increase in blood histamine levels after EIU and have suggested this as the cause of the urticaria. Others have suggested a generalized hypersensitivity to acetylcholine as the mechanism.

Treatment involves avoidance of exercise in hot, humid conditions. Pretreatment with antihistamines such as hydroxyzine may also be effective.

## EXERCISE-INDUCED ANAPHYLAXIS

Exercise-induced anaphylaxis (EIAn) is rare, but it is the most serious form of exercise-induced allergic reaction. It is characterized initially by pruritus, flushing, and erythema. It then progresses to urticaria (large 10 to 15 mm lesions); laryngospasm; angioedema of the face, hands, and feet; and finally vascular collapse. Gastrointestinal symptoms—such as colic, nausea, and diarrhea—may also occur.

EIAn is usually provoked by high intensity exercise, but it does not consistently occur with every exercise exposure. Risk factors include a personal or family history of atopy, exercising in hot and humid environments, and preexercise ingestion of food. The most common foods associated with EIAn are aspirin products, caffeine, shellfish, and celery.

EIAn is a unique form of physical allergy and is distinct from EIB and EIU. It is associated with mast cell degranulation, and high levels of histamine are seen following an episode. The trigger mechanism is unclear. There is some evidence of a genetic predisposition.

Treatment of an acute collapse consists of epinephrine, oxygen, fluids, antihistamines, and general supportive measures. Antihistamines may be

---

### PREVENTION OF EXERCISE-INDUCED ANAPHYLAXIS

Carry an epinephrine kit.
Exercise with a "buddy" trained in the use of epinephrine.
Decrease the intensity of the exercise.
Avoid exercising in hot, humid conditions.
Avoid eating before exercising.
Stop exercising at the first sign of flushing, generalized warmth, or
    pruritus.

partially effective and are recommended for prophylactic and acute therapy. Individuals with a history of EIAn should carry an epinephrine kit and exercise with a "buddy" trained in the use of epinephrine. These patients should also decrease the intensity of the exercise; avoid exercising in hot, humid conditions; avoid eating 4 to 6 hours before exercising; and stop exercising at the first sign of flushing, generalized warmth, or pruritus. (See the box on p. 34.)

## SUMMARY

Allergic reactions can occur in athletic individuals as a result of exposure to common allergens, or they may be exercise-induced. EIB is a common cause of exercise intolerance and can be controlled in the majority of people. Nonpharmacologic and pharmacologic treatment modalities are successful. Care must be taken to select medications approved by the IOC when treating athletes competing in IOC-USOC sponsored events. EIU is a bothersome clinical entity that can be controlled using antihistamines. EIAn is rare but potentially fatal; patients who experience this reaction must be properly educated in prevention techniques.

### Bibliography

Anderson SD: Exercise-induced asthma: the state of the art, *Chest* 87(suppl 5):191s-195s, 1985.

Belcher NG, Murdoch R, Dalton N et al: Circulating concentrations of histamine, neutrophil chemotactic activity, and catecholamines during the refractory period in exercise-induced asthma, *J Allergy Clin Immunol* 81:100-110, 1988.

Bergmann K-Ch: Sports and allergy, *Int J Sports Med* 12(suppl 1):16s-18s, 1991.

Bermann BA, Ross RN: Exercise-induced bronchospasm: is it a unique clinical entity? *Ann Allergy Asthma Immunol* 65:81, 1990.

Blumenthal MN: Sports-aggravated allergies: how to treat and prevent the symptoms, *Physician Sports Med* 18:52-66, 1990.

Briner WW, Sheffer AL: Introduction: exercise and allergy, *Med Sci Sports Exerc* 24:843-844, 1992.

Crimi E, Balbo A, Milanese M et al: Airway inflammation and occurrence of delayed bronchoconstriction in exercise-induced asthma, *Am Rev Respir Dis* 146:507-512, 1992.

Eggleston PA, Rosenthal SA, Anderson R et al: Guidelines for the methodology of exercise challenge testing of asthmatics, *J Allergy Clin Immunol* 64:642-645, 1979.

Godfrey S: Introduction: symposium on special problems and management of allergic athletes, *J Allergy Clin Immunol* 73:630-633, 1984.

Gorevic PD, Kaplan AP: The physical urticarias, *Int J Dermatol* 19:417-435, 1980.

Holgate ST, Finnerty JP: Antihistamines in asthma, *J Allergy Clin Immunol* 83:537-547, 1989.

Huftel MA, Gaddy JN, Busse WW: Finding and managing asthma in competitive athletes, *J Respir Dis* 12:1110-1122, 1991.

Kaplan AP, Gray LL, Shaff RE et al: In vivo studies of mediator release in cold urticaria and cholinergic urticaria, *J Allergy Clin Immunol* 55:394-402, 1985.

Kaplan AP, Natbony SF, Tawil AP et al: Exercise-induced anaphylaxis as a manifestation of cholinergic urticaria, *J Allergy Clin Immunol* 68:319-324, 1981.

Katz RM: Exercise-induced asthma/other allergic reactions in the athlete, *Allergy Proc* 10:203-208, 1989.

Katz RM: Rhinitis in the athlete, *J Allergy Clin Immunol* 73:708-711, 1984.

Kobayashi RH, Mellion MB: Exercise-induced asthma, anaphylaxis, and urticaria, *Prim Care* 18:809-831, 1991.

Kuzemko JA: Anaphylactic syndrome induced by exercise, *Practitioner* 230:209, 1986.

Kyle JM, Walker SL, Hanshaw JR et al: Exercise-induced bronchospasm in the young athlete: guidelines for routine screening and initial management, *Med Sci Sports Exerc* 24:856-859, 1992.

Lewis JP, Lieberman G, Treadwell J et al: Exercise-induced urticaria, angioedema and anaphylactoid episodes, *J Allergy Clin Immunol* 68:432-437, 1981.

Longley S, Panush RS: Familial exercise-induced anaphylaxis, *Ann Allergy* 58:257-259, 1987.

Mahler DA: Exercise-induced asthma, *Med Sci Sports Exerc* 25:554-561, 1993.

McFadden ER Jr: Exercise-induced asthma: assessment of current etiologic concepts, *Chest* 91(suppl 1):151s-157s, 1987.

Mellion MB, Kobayashi RH: Exercise-induced asthma, *Am Fam Physician* 45:2671-2677, 1992.

Obata T, Kishida M, Okuma M et al: A case of exercise-induced anaphylaxis: evidence of an association with the complement system, *Acta Paediatr Jpn* 31:340-345, 1989.

Sheffer AL, Austen KF: Exercise-induced anaphylaxis, *J Allergy Clin Immunol* 73:699-703, 1984.

Sheffer AL, Tong AKF, Murphy RA et al: Exercise-induced anaphylaxis: a serious form of physical allergy associated with mast cell degranulation, *J Allergy Clin Immunol* 75:479-484, 1985.

Silvers WS: Exercise-induced allergies: the role of histamine release, *Ann Allergy* 68:58-63, 1992.

Silvers WS: The skier's nose: a model of cold induced rhinorrhea, *Ann Allergy* 67:32-36, 1991.

United States Olympic Committee Drug Education and Doping Control Progam: *Guide to banned medications*, Colorado Springs, Colo, 1993, The Committee.

Virant FS: Exercise-induced bronchospasm: epidemiology, pathophysiology, and therapy, *Med Sci Sports Exerc* 24:851-855, 1992.

# Chapter 4

# Dental trauma

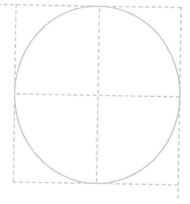

John F. Wisniewski

## GENERAL CONSIDERATIONS

The human dentition serves four basic functions: (1) mastication (chewing), (2) speech (uttering phonetic sounds), (3) aesthetics, and (4) support of the overlying soft tissues (lips, cheeks, etc.). Each type of tooth has a main purpose. Incisors, located in the front of the arch, are primarily used in cutting. Canines, situated at the corner of the arch, serve mainly in ripping or tearing. Premolars, positioned midway from the corner toward the posterior segment of the arch, assist in the combination effect of ripping-tearing plus mashing-grinding. Molars, found in the most posterior segment of the arch, aid primarily in mashing or grinding. Nature has developed and shaped each tooth group for a specific role. Incisors have a sharp and narrow cutting edge (via a labiolingual dimension); canines tend to be long and pointed, with lengthy roots firmly embedded in the bone; premolars have sharper cusp tips than molars and wider edges than canines; and, lastly, molars have a greater number of cusps, more-rounded cusp tips, and a broader occlusal (biting) surface than premolars.

Depending on the shape, number of roots, and position on the arch, some teeth are more susceptible to fracture and displacement trauma than are others. Anterior teeth, such as incisors and canines, have wider working edges or biting surfaces (via a mesiodistal or sidewise direction) in comparison with their "necks" or cervical line areas. Additionally, the height of the crown of an anterior tooth is longer than that of a posterior tooth. Finally, because anterior teeth are located toward the front of the mouth, they are more susceptible to direct trauma. In view of these anatomic considerations, anterior teeth tend to demonstrate a wide variety of fractures to their crowns as compared with those of posterior teeth. When a blow is received to the anterior segment, the force frequently fractures the edges of an incisor or establishes a fulcrum at the neck of the tooth, thus breaking off the crown. These three aforementioned factors, combined with root morphology, allow one to better understand root fractures and displacement trauma.

In general, posterior teeth—especially maxillary first premolars, maxillary molars, and mandibular molars—are multirooted, whereas anterior teeth are single-rooted. Maxillary first premolars and mandibular molars have two roots; the maxillary molars contain three. The cross-sectional shapes of anterior roots tend to be circular or rounded triangles; their shapes lengthwise are straight and conical. In comparison, cross-sectional areas of posterior tooth roots demonstrate wider buccolingual or buccopalatal dimensions, in addition to containing various depressions or concavities at significant locations. Mandibular molar roots are slightly curved; maxillary molar roots tend to diverge as they enter the alveolar bone. Finally, the buccal and palatal-lingual bony plates that support the teeth are narrower in the anterior area than they are in the posterior area. Combining root morphology with the aforementioned anatomic considerations gives the clinician the knowledge to better understand why there are fewer root fractures in posterior teeth and why anterior teeth are more prone to displacement trauma related to their alveolar sockets than are posterior teeth. Essentially, posterior teeth are more firmly embedded and supported by bone than are anterior teeth.

## ANATOMY AND HISTOLOGY

The oral cavity is composed of two parts: the upper jaw and the lower jaw. The upper jaw, or maxillary arch, is stationary. This arch is attached to the cranium via the temporal bones, frontal bones, zygomatic bones, and nasal bones. The lower jaw, or mandibular arch, is the movable segment. Except for the bite established by the dentition, there is no other interaction between the maxilla and the mandible. In fact, complaints concerning an alteration in this bite are helpful tools in determining whether a patient has incurred a fracture of the mandible or of the maxillary arch. The temporomandibular joint, connecting the mandible to the temporal bone, is the only joint in the body possessing the ability to move in both a hinge and a gliding motion. When opening for approximately the first 10 mm, rotation of the condyles occurs in the sagittal plane. As this distance continues to increase, the condyles begin to slide down anteriorly over the articular tubercle of the temporal bone.

Each arch is divided into halves, which are known as quadrants. Thus four quadrants comprise an entire mouth. The primary dentition (deciduous or "baby" teeth) contains 20 teeth. Each quadrant consists of two incisors, one canine ("eye" tooth), and two molars. The permanant dentition ("adult" teeth) incorporates 32 teeth, or eight teeth per quadrant. These teeth include two incisors, one canine, two premolars, and three molars (Fig. 4-1). Third molars are commonly referred to as "wisdom" teeth. A mixed dentition occurs when any combination of primary and permanent teeth exists in an individual's mouth at a given point in time.

A precise lettering and numbering system facilitates communication among dentists, as well as between dentists and dental paraprofessionals. The most often used system is the Universal system. Deciduous teeth are designated by a capital letter of the alphabet (*A* to *T*); permanent teeth receive a number (*1* to *32*) (Fig. 4-1). In each case the first tooth to be labeled is that which normally is located in the most posterior portion of the right maxillary arch. The lettering-numbering continues anteriorly across the upper arch to the upper left quadrant, then drops down to the mandibular left quadrant and proceeds again anteriorly across the lower arch until the last molar in the mandibular right quadrant has been identified. Thus the deciduous right maxillary second molar is identified as *A*; the deciduous left maxillary molar as *J*; the deciduous left mandibular second molar as *K*; and, finally, the deciduous right mandibular second molar as *T*. In the permanent dentition, the upper right third molar is labeled as *1*; the upper left third molar as *16*; the lower left third molar as *17*; and, lastly, the lower right third molar as *32*. The letters and numbers in-between those listed here correspond to the appropiate remaining teeth in the dentition.

The alveolar bone (alveolus) of maxillary  and mandibular arches houses the dentition. Each individual tooth is located in an alveolar socket and retained there by the periodontal ligament. Displacement traumatic injuries that occur and alter the gross relationship between a tooth and an alveolar socket also violate the integrity of the periodontal ligament on a cellular level (Fig. 4-2).

A tooth contains four types of tissues: (1) enamel, (2) cementum, (3) dentin, and (4) pulp. The first three—enamel, cementum, and dentin—are hard tissues. The last—pulp—is soft tissue. Each tooth has two main portions: (1) the crown, which is the portion of the tooth covered by enamel; and (2) the root, which is the portion covered by cementum. The tip of the root is called the apex. The junction of the crown to the root, or cementum to enamel, is known as the cementoenamel junction (CEJ) or cervical line. The bulk of the tooth is composed of dentin. The innermost layer, which is solely soft tissue, is called the pulp. The pulpal tissue furnishes the arterial, venous, and nerve supplies to the tooth. This tissue travels through the dentin via odontoblastic processes. Ultimately these processes anastomose at the dentoenamel junction (DEJ) or end at the root surface.

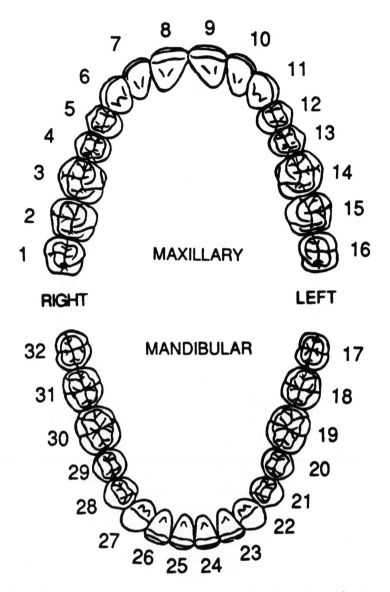

**Fig. 4-1.** Universal numbering system: permanent dentition. (Drawn by Dr. Perng-Ru Liu.)

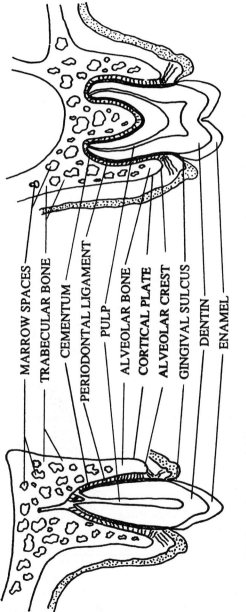

POSTERIOR TOOTH

ANTERIOR TOOTH

MARROW SPACES
TRABECULAR BONE
CEMENTUM
PERIODONTAL LIGAMENT
PULP
ALVEOLAR BONE
CORTICAL PLATE
ALVEOLAR CREST
GINGIVAL SULCUS
DENTIN
ENAMEL

**Fig. 4-2.** Anatomy of the teeth and supporting tissues. (Drawn by Dr. Perng-Ru Liu.)

Traumatic injuries of the oral cavity may involve the soft tisue, the hard tissue, or a combination of both. Having reviewed general information about the oral cavity and teeth, as well as the basic anatomy and histology, the clinician is now better equipped to understand dental trauma.

## SOFT TISSUE INJURIES

Soft tissue injuries can occur to many aspects of the oral cavity, including the following areas:

1. Skin or face
2. Lips
3. Cheeks
4. Labial mucosa (underside of lips)
5. Buccal mucosa (underside of cheeks)
6. Tongue
7. Floor of mouth
8. Hard palate
9. Soft palate
10. Gingiva (gums)

Soft tissue injuries can usually be classsified as one of four types:
1. *Contusion*: a blunt trauma wound; usually the overlying tissues are bruised.
2. *Abrasion*: denuded epidermis injury; its surface is a raw, bleeding area.
3. *Laceration*: a superficial or deep tear of soft tissue; it may be inflicted by a sharp object.
4. *Penetration*: a perforation wound; it is inflicted by a small-diameter object that penetrates the tissue.

There are three principles of treatment for soft tissue injuries: (1) irrigation, (2) immobilization, and (3) coverage. A thorough lavage  and a conservative debridement of the wound are essential to prevent secondary infection. Meticulous suturing techniques aid in attaining primary wound closure. Lip lacerations that cross the vermilion border are of particular concern. While suturing, care must be taken to reestablish the alignment of this border exactly, lest a noticeable scar should develop. Tooth fracture, in combination with a lip laceration, necessitates careful debridement and inspection of the wound. Often, diagnostic radiographs are taken of a lip laceration. This procedure helps to determine whether or not portions of a tooth are embedded in the soft tissue. If primary closure is attained without removing these tooth fragments, then these particles will not resorb, but will only serve to become a nidus for infection. On occasion, after irrigating and suturing the lip wound, coverage is sometimes necessary. When such is the case, this final aspect is difficult to negotiate and necessitates patient cooperation to maintain the protective barrier. Before dismissal, the patient should be evaluated for tetanus inoculation, as well as for prophylactic antibiotic coverage.

Although the discussion thus far has focused on evaluating superficial soft tissue trauma, the clinician must be aware of the underlying anatomic structures. The oral cavity contains a complex network of nerve, venous, and arterial supplies. Additionally, salivary glands and ducts lie directly below the floor of the mouth (lingual and submandibular salivary glands), as well as within the cheeks and lateral to the maxillary second molars (parotid glands). When trauma occurs, violation of the nerve or blood supply may be obvious. However, a severed salivary duct may be less apparent. Care must be taken not to suture a duct closed. If a duct is sutured, a clinical swelling will begin to occur before and during mealtime. The gland will continue to secrete saliva, but there is no outlet. Symptoms tend to mimic those of a salivary duct obstruction (e.g., a salivary stone).

## HARD TISSUE INJURIES

### TOOTH INJURIES

Accidents that produce traumatic injuries to the teeth themselves are often accompanied by hemorrhage, swelling, and laceration of tissue. Such injuries tend to frighten people and therefore may complicate the examination. Dental trauma has been described by two systems, the Ellis and the World Health Organization systems. These two classifications have been referred to extensively and provide the basis for most systems used in textbooks and articles. A more practical classification system, which can be used by nondental health care professionals when communicating with dentists, simply divides tooth injuries into two groups. These groups emerge based on which portion of a tooth sustains the injury—for instance, the crown of the tooth or the root of the tooth.

Injuries to the crown of a tooth can be evaluated according to the following categories:

1. *Class I fracture:* fracture of the enamel portion only
2. *Class II fracture:* fracture line includes dentin, but no pulp exposure
3. *Class III fracture:* fracture of the crown with exposed pulp

Root fractures are the second major category of tooth injuries. These fractures can occur at or below the cervical line. A root fracture is classified as either a cervical-third fracture, a middle-third fracture, or an apical-third fracture.

When a tooth has been fractured or is suspected of being fractured, professional examination is imperative. The clinical treatment is determined by a good medical history, a history of the accident, and a careful clinical and radiologic examination. Radiographs are often necessary to determine the severity of the fracture and also serve as a baseline for future observation of the tooth. In addition, broken pieces of the tooth frequently become embedded in soft tissue (e.g., the lips) and are best located by a radiograph. In general, "the larger the fracture, the more severe the problem." An athlete who sustains a class I fracture to an incisor usually expresses more concerns about the appearance than complaints about any symptoms. This type of fracture is confined to enamel only. A fracture of this degree involves the dentin portion of a tooth. Tooth pain is usually not present; however, a patient may state that the fractured portion is sharp and is irritating his or her lips or tongue.

In addition to concerns about appearance and surface roughness, an individual sustaining a class II fracture may complain about sensitivity to cold. This is due to the direct communication of the pulp through the dentin via the odontoblastic processes. A fracture of this degree involves the dentin portion of a tooth. With both class I and II fractures, there is no restriction regarding return to play. Follow-up care and evaluation by a dentist should be scheduled immediately following the athletic competition.

An athlete exhibiting a class III fracture usually has significant pain in addition to any combination of the clinical symptoms that are associated with class I and II fractures. In this type of fracture, the pulp is directly injured and exposed. The tooth may demonstrate a red spot or may bleed. This is because the pulp contains the blood supply, as well as the nerve to the tooth. Ideally, return to play should be postponed until the athlete has received an examination and treatment by a dentist. With regard to class I, II, or III tooth fractures, the prognosis for the athlete retaining an involved tooth as part of his or her existing dentition is excellent. However, advanced treatment, such as root canal therapy, is frequently required in the treatment of class III fractures.

The prognosis for root fractures is not quite as optimistic. In general, the closer the fracture is to the cervical line, the poorer the prognosis. If a root fracture appears likely, the athlete should not be allowed to return to play. Clinical symptoms may range from no symptoms or a dull ache, to extreme pain. In the case of a suspected root fracture, as well as a class III fracture, ideally a dental evaluation should be immediate or as soon as possible following the injury.

## TOOTH-TO-BONE INJURIES

In addition to tooth injuries, a second category of hard tissue injuries involves the violation of the tooth-to-bone relationship. These types of injuries involve the displacement of a tooth in relation to the alveolar socket. This group includes the following injuries:

1. Tooth luxation: loosening and displacement of the tooth in relationship to the athlete's existing arch form. Frequently this type of

injury is accompanied by fracture and comminution (fragmentation) of the alveolar socket. Often the blow comes from an anteroposterior direction.

A complaint often expressed by the athlete is that his or her "bite is off" or that, "I am not biting right." If a dentist is not present, the team physician or a member of the athletic training staff may feel comfortable in diagnosing the injury. Bilateral digital palpation will lead to an assessment of the tooth arch deformation. If possible, the clinician should gently guide the tooth back into alignment. Most often the athlete will determine the success of repositioning via visual examination, as well as by closure of his or her dentition. Should the treatment be successful, follow-up evaluation by a dentist may be scheduled at the earliest convenience. The athlete should be advised to maintain a soft-food diet, with no excessive biting to the injured area until he or she has been examined by a dentist.

If, however, if the tooth is extremely mobile—for instance, a 3 mm or greater displacement in a labiopalatal-labiolingual direction—evaluation by a dentist immediately following the athletic event should be scheduled. A conservative physician will not allow the athlete to return to play.

2. Tooth intrusion: displacement of the tooth into the alveolar bone; it is accompanied by fracture of the alveolar socket. The force of the blow involved in this type of injury usually is directed along an inferior vector to a superior vector. An intrusion is a very violent injury on a cellular level. Not only does a direct fracture occur within that alveolar socket, but periodontal ligament cells are crushed, torn, and abraded in addition to bone marrow spaces being crushed or compressed.

Following an intrusion injury the damage has already been done. The conservative team physician will not allow the athlete to return to play. Caution should be advised because this injury is extremely painful. The athlete may be distracted by the pain, thus predisposing him or her to further injuries—as well as subpar performance—if allowed to continue to play. The athlete should receive a clinical and radiographic examination by a dentist as soon as possible.

3. Tooth extrusion: a partial displacement of the tooth out of its socket. The directions of the forces are usually at an angle coming from superior reference points to the inferior reference points. The blow usually engages the tooth below the height of contour, thus catching it and driving it out of the socket. In this case the nerve, arterial supply, venous supply, and periodontal ligaments are torn.

Similar to those for a tooth luxation injury, recommendations should include a soft-food diet, with no excessive biting to the injured area until the athlete has been examined by a dentist. However, in addition to bilateral digital palpation in assessing the injury and realigning the tooth, instructing the athlete to bite down on folded cotton gauze also may be helpful in repositioning the tooth back up into its socket. The athlete should not be allowed to return to play and should be examined by a dentist immediately.

4. Tooth avulsion: an exarticulation or complete displacement of the tooth out of its socket. The direction of the blow and the anatomic disturbances parallel those of a tooth extrusion injury. However, in this case replantation of the tooth must be addressed.

To understand the concept of tooth replantation, the anatomy of the avulsed tooth must be discussed (Fig. 4-3). When a tooth is avulsed from its socket, the periodontal ligament—which retains the tooth in the alveolar socket—is torn; some portions of the ligament remain in the bony socket while other segments remain attached to the tooth. The portion of the ligament that remains in the socket maintains viability with no additional treatment. However, the questionable area (and that of concern) is the portion of the ligament that is still left attached to the tooth. Maintaining the morphology and physiology of

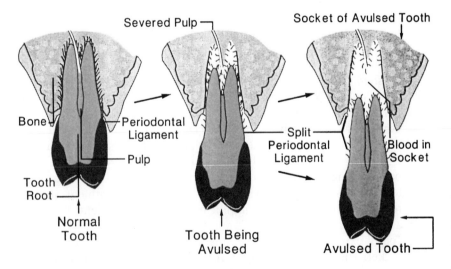

**Fig. 4-3.** Anatomy of tooth avulsion. (From Krasner PR: Treatment of tooth avulsion in the emergency department: appropriate storage and transport media, *Am J Emerg Med* 8:351-355, 1990.)

the periodontal ligament cells is essential if a replanted tooth is to be retained for life.

There are three stages of avulsed tooth treatment:

Stage I: preservation, storage, and transportation to a dentist

Stage II: emergency dental treatment by a dentist

Stage III: follow-up dental treatment

If the attending team physician feels comfortable replanting the tooth then this should be done immediately. Before replantation, the tooth should be rinsed off with a pH-balanced preserving solution or sterile saline and guided back into its socket by having the athlete bite on gauze. At no time should the crown or root be scraped, scrubbed, or treated with disinfectant chemicals or detergents. Any of the aforementioned would cause periodontal ligament cell death. Visual inspection of the athlete and confirmation from him or her that the bite, or occlusion, is normal are two initial checks to determine if the tooth has been successfully "fitted" back into the dental arch. If this procedure is accomplished within 15 to 30 minutes following the injury, there is a 90% chance that the tooth will be retained. Since time is critical, the athlete should not be allowed to return to play but should be examined by a dentist immediately; the tooth should be replanted as soon as possible.

Obviously when treating an athlete with an avulsed tooth, "time is of the essence." The sooner the tooth can be replanted, the better (Fig. 4-4). However, if the time frame extends beyond 30 minutes, or

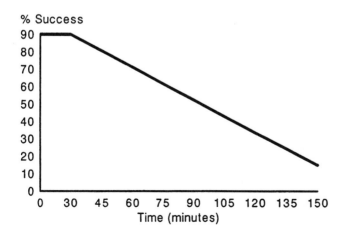

**Fig. 4-4.** Avulsed tooth success rate versus extraoral time. (From Krasner PR: Treatment of tooth avulsion in the emergency department: appropriate storage and transport media, *Am J Emerg Med* 8:351-355, 1990.)

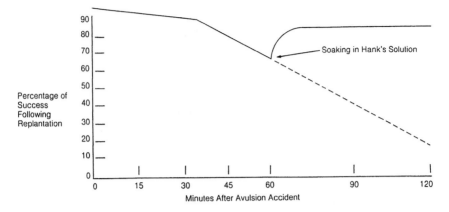

**Fig. 4-5.** The success rate of replanted teeth: soaking versus nonsoaking. (From Krasner PR: Management of tooth avulsion in the school setting, *J Sch Nurs* 8:20-26, 1992.)

if the physician chooses not to replant immediately, the clinician needs to further understand the critical concepts underlying stage I. The periodontal ligament cells that remain attached to the tooth must not be crushed; and normal cell composition, morphology, and physiology must be maintained. Immediate replantation, as previously discussed, creates such an environment. However, when this is not an option, what are the criteria for storage media and methods of transportation?

The worst possible storage-transportation medium is a dry medium such as a tissue or gauze. Drying out the periodontal ligaments causes rapid cell death. Equally destructive is allowing the tooth to "air dry" or soaking the avulsed tooth in tap water, which disrupts the cell morphology and will ultimately cause lysis of the periodontal ligament cells. Sterile saline may be used if the avulsed tooth is not soaked in it for more than 1 hour. However, sterile saline lacks the nutrients that are necessary to replenish those used by the normal metabolic processes of the periodontal ligament cells.

Saliva can be used as a storage medium for short periods of time, but if it is used for a time period longer than 1 hour, cellular damage will occur. Additionally, contamination by the bacteria from the normal oral flora can be destructive and complicate treatment. The saliva can be collected in a container or the tooth can be placed under the athlete's tongue. Age, presence of intraoral bleeding, and consciousness of the player—as well as the mental composure of the athlete—all help determine whether or not using saliva is a viable option. Cold milk is an acceptable storage medium, but it is not always available on site. The best storage media are pH-balanced culture fluids such as Hank's solution or Eagle's medium. Both are biocompatible with periodontal ligament cells and can keep the cells viable for 4 to 12 hours. These solutions do not need to be refrigerated, have a long shelf-life, and can therefore be made part of an emergency kit. These fluids can rejuvenate the degenerated periodontal ligament cells and maintain a success rate for replantation of over 90% when an avulsed tooth is soaked in either fluid for 30 minutes (Fig. 4-5).

Once an acceptable storage medium has been established, transportation media guidelines need to be considered. The tooth should not be handled by the root portion. Touching the root surface may cause crushing of the periodontal ligament cells, leading to potential cell death. Thus the manner in which a tooth is transported can significantly affect the success rate for replantation.

In general, the ideal transport container should possess the following characteristics:

1. Break-resistant
2. Nontoxic
3. Easy to use
4. Soft inner walls
5. Tightly fitting cap
6. Sterile
7. Protects tooth during transport
8. Permits debris on the tooth to be washed off
9. Facilitates easy, atraumatic removal of the tooth
10. Air-tight and leak-proof

At the site of an athletic injury, the transportation medium that is ultimately chosen probably will not meet several of these criteria. Additionally, an athlete may have also incurred a more severe and/or life threatening injury. In that case—according to a triage system—the oral injury, and especially the care of the avulsed tooth, would receive the least amount of attention (and rightly so). Thus the success rate of replantation in either of the above cases would be compromised. However, this is not a reflection on the attending health care professional, but rather it is solely an outcome related to the prevailing circumstances.

The result of these conditions can easily be altered by incorporating Save•A•Tooth, the emergency tooth preserving system, into a physician's medical bag or a trainer's emergency kit. The Save•A•Tooth system (Fig. 4-6) is small, very economical, and meets the ideal standards for transportation and storage media. It contains sterile pH-balanced preserving solution (Hank's solution), is break resistant, and has a screw-on cap. It has a suspension device inside the container that holds the tooth securely during transport. This protects the tooth and simultaneously permits the washing of the tooth. A handle on this basket allows the dentist to easily remove the tooth from the container without damaging the tooth. Storage and transport in this system will safely preserve the tooth for up to 12 hours.

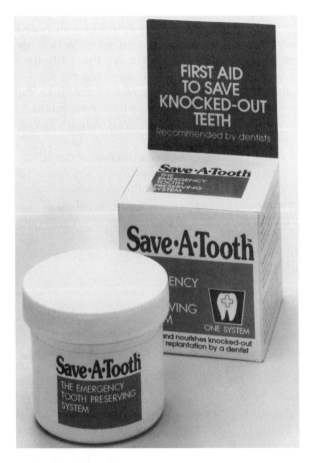

**Fig. 4-6.** Save•A•Tooth: the emergency tooth preserving system. (Courtesy of Biological Rescue Products, Inc.)

## BONE INJURIES

The maxillofacial complex is composed of seven bones—two of which are single bones, and five are paired. The single bones are the mandible and vomer; the paired bones are the maxilla, zygomatic, nasal, lacrimal, and palatine. Injuries to the maxillofacial complex may involve only one bone or any combination of these bones. The primary goals in treating injuries to the face are to restore function of facial structures and to restore appearance. The abundant blood supply to the maxillofacial complex predisposes facial wounds to good healing, thus facilitating the attainment of the two goals of treatment.

The initial consideration when treating an athlete with a facial injury is the evaluation and maintenance of airway, breathing, and circulation. Prevention or treatment of hemorrhagic shock, evaluation for loss of consciousness, early and thorough physical examination, and continuous neurologic assessment are essential standards for optimal care for all such injuries.

Suspected injuries to the maxillofacial complex require clinical, as well as radiologic, evaluation. Palpation and intraoral examination aid in the detection of skeletal injuries. Malocclusion is a classic finding in mandibular fractures with displacement, but it may also occur in midface and maxillary injuries. Ecchymosis in the floor of the mouth is almost pathognomonic of a mandibular fracture. Mucosal ecchymosis near the zygomatic buttress occurs in fractures of the zygoma and in midface fractures. A "gagged bite" is the common finding in midface fractures with retrodisplacement of the maxillary segment. Finally, every athlete who has a midface fracture should receive an eye examination and a simple test of visual acuity.

If possible, radiographs of the face should be taken immediately. The occipitomental (Waters) view assists in evaluating the maxilla, the zygoma, and the frontal sinuses; oblique views are helpful in examining the mandible and lower third of the face; a panorex, which involves a radiograph being taken circumferentially around the athlete's face, is useful in determining the extent of mandibular injuries. Lastly, a Towne's view of the mandibular condyles aids in the detection of condylar fractures.

## CONCLUSION

As has been stated previously, and in general following a dental or oral injury, "time is of the essence." The sooner that the athlete can receive an examination by a dentist, the better. Dental professionals who are capable of treating tooth and tooth-to-bone injuries include general dentists, pediatric (children's) dentists, and endodontists (root canal specialists). Oral surgeons should be consulted regarding any suspected bone injuries. Team physicians and trainers should have a list of on-call dentists or, preferably, a specific dentist who is affiliated with their athletic program or team. Additionally, nondental health care professionals should be aware of the hospitals, emergency rooms, and trauma centers in their immediate area.

Important information to be obtained includes answers to the following questions:

1. Does the hospital have a dentist or oral surgeon on call?
2. Does the hospital have a general practice dental residency program?
   a. Is the dental resident on beeper-call? *or*
   b. Is the dental resident in-house, or hospital-based?

Having answers to these questions will allow the physician and trainer to know in advance where an athlete will be sent if a dental-oral injury occurs. Emergency dental care can be given to the athlete more quickly if a team dentist is "on staff" or if the dental resources of the hospital in the immediate vicinity have been previously investigated. Finally, it is important to telephone ahead to the hospital emergency room or dental office—especially in the case of an avulsed tooth—since time is a critical factor. This allows a dentist time to set up an emergency operatory, adjust the patient schedule, and render emergency care in an efficient manner. Similarly, a hospital can call in the appropriate personnel to give immediate care to the athlete on arrival.

## Acknowledgment

The author wishes to thank Ms. Katrina Fowler for typing the manuscript of this chapter.

## Dedication

This chapter is dedicated to my parents, John and Mary Wisniewski, for their sacrifice in providing me the opportunity to attain an education.

## Bibliography

Ash MM Jr: *Wheeler's dental anatomy, physiology, and occlusion,* ed 7, Philadelphia, 1993, WB Saunders.

Clark JW, editor: *Clinical dentistry,* vol 3, Hagerstown, Md, 1978, Harper & Row.

Clinical symposia: maxillofacial injuries, *Ciba Found Symp,* vol 33, 1981.

Ellis GE, Davey KW: *The classification and treatment of injuries to the teeth of children,* ed 5, Chicago, 1970, Mosby–Year Book.

Krasner P: The athletic trainer's role in saving avulsed teeth, *Athletic Training* 24:139-142, 1989.

Kruger GO, editor: *Textbook of oral surgery,* ed 4, St Louis, 1974, Mosby–Year Book.

Rowe NL, Williams JL, editors: *Maxillofacial injuries,* vol 1, London, 1985, Churchill Livingstone.

World Health Organization: *Application of the international classification of diseases to dentistry and stomatology,* ed 7, ICD-DA, Geneva, 1978, The Organization.

**Chapter 5**

# Chest injuries

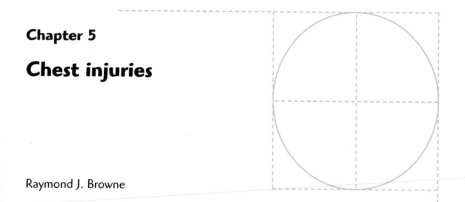

Raymond J. Browne

## CARDIAC CONTUSIONS

There are several potential causes for a cardiac contusion. The most common cause is a direct blow to the chest. This results in a compression of the heart between the sternum and the thoracic spine. A less common cause is a contrecoup injury that occurs during deceleration. The mechanism involved with this type of injury is similar to the mechanism that occurs with a cerebral injury. An example is an athlete who is running fast and is suddenly hit directly, so that his or her heart proceeds anteriorly against the sternum and then swings posteriorly against the thoracic spine. A rare cause for a contusion to the myocardium is a sudden increase in intrathoracic pressure.

The most common complaint of an athlete with a cardiac contusion is chest pain. The athlete may also complain of pleuritic pain that is aggravated by twisting or coughing, and is actually eased by sitting or leaning forward. A physical exam of the athlete is remarkable, usually finding tachycardia and tachypnea. The athlete may also appear diaphoretic, and may complain of nausea and experience vomiting. With the development of fluid in the pericardium the exam may be remarkable for muffled heart sounds and a narrowing pulse pressure. (The pulse pressure is the difference between the systolic and the diastolic values in mm Hg.) Pulsus paradoxus (e.g., the inspiratory diminution in arterial pressure exceeds 10 mm Hg) and intrajugular venous distention with Kussmaul's sign (when the inspiratory venous pressure remains steady or increases) indicate the potential for cardiac tamponade. An audible friction rub and a rapid Y descent when assessing the jugular venous patterns are suggestive of constrictive pericarditis.

If radiographic facilities are available, then it is important to obtain a chest x-ray. This will allow the physician to determine whether there is a sternal fracture or rib fractures that compound the severity of the trauma to the chest. A "water bottle" cardiac silhouette finding is usually indicative of a worsening hemorrhage into the pericardium. The presence of this sign on a posteroanterior view of the chest mandates immediate triage to a tertiary care facility or an attempted pericardiocentesis if the athlete's condition is deteriorating rapidly.

Electrocardiographic changes are evident in approximately 50% of cases of significant chest trauma. The most common finding is a T wave flattening or T wave inversion in one or more leads. The next most frequent change is a slight ST depression. Localized ST segment elevation is rare. Pathologic Q waves are indicative of actual damage to the myocardium. Despite definitive damage to the myocardium, the electrocardiogram (ECG) may be normal. Since the right ventricle is located anteriorly, it is particularly vulnerable to any anterior trauma. Damage to the right ventricle may be silent on the ECG since depolarization is frequently overshadowed by thicker ventricular septum and the left ventricular free wall. ECG changes usually occur within hours after the trauma, but frequently they are delayed for approximately 48 hours and may not appear for up to 5 days after the chest injury. These changes, if they are not indicative of actual damage to the myocardium, usually resolve in 4 to 30 days. In addition, one may also see transient abnormalities of conduction.

Treatment of a cardiac contusion usually involves hospitalization with further evaluation inclusive of cardiac monitoring. Creatine phosphokinase (CPK) and MB enzymes are often drawn to support the suspicion of trauma to the myocardium. However, this is considered an isolated test and not diagnostic of a cardiac contusion. One of the initial tests that should be performed is an echocardiogram. This test is important for assessing the wall motion of different chambers. This is also a good means for determining the presence of a pericardial effusion, a ruptured septum, or an aneurysm. A technetium pyrophosphate scan is useful when there are nonspecific ECG changes. This scan is usually positive 12 to 24 hours after the cardiac trauma; it may revert to normal after 5 days. However, the persistence of activity with the technetium pyrophosphate scan may be indicative of aneurysm formation. If the aforementioned tests still leave some doubt about the wall motion and function of the myocardium, then a cardiac catheterization should be performed to assess the presence of any coronary arterial lesions and to quantify the presence of any structural cardiac lesions.

Treatment usually involves monitoring the heart for the first several days to make sure that there is no evidence of any arrhythmias secondary to the trauma to the myocardium. The patient also should be placed on complete bed rest for several days, with a gradual increase in activities over a 1- to 2-week period as tolerated. During the first several weeks after the cardiac contusion the athlete should avoid heavy isometric activity. The concern here is the possible predisposition to arrhythmias in delayed myocardial rupture.

## COMMOTIO CORDIS

*Commotio cordis* is Latin for "commotion of the heart." This usually occurs secondary to impact of the anterior chest wall. It is theorized that this trauma to the heart results in disruption of electrical conduction in the heart, which leads to cardiac arrhythmias, ventricular fibrillation, and ventricular asystole. The clinical scenario usually involves a healthy young individual who incurs a blunt impact to the anterior chest wall, collapses suddenly, and becomes unresponsive.

Since there is a high incidence of ventricular fibrillation, it is recommended that immediate treatment proceed with a precordial thump. It is then important to obtain adequate ventilatory support to lessen the myocardial acidosis, which causes myocardial suppression and subsequent reduction in cardiac output. If there is no response, cardiopulmonary resuscitation (CPR) should be conducted and continued until the athlete is triaged to the nearest emergency room.

Unfortunately, despite immediate CPR and adequate ventilatory support, the survival rate is extremely low. Thus prevention becomes more important in averting this potential catastrophe. For instance, in a sport such as football athletes should be instructed to avoid a direct blow to the anterior chest wall from the ball by catching it in front of the body with the hands. In addition, it is recommended that the velocity of impact loading be reduced with proper padding and improved chest musculature. It is also important to educate athletes. This is usually done with agility and coordination drills to prevent a potentially lethal impact to the chest.

## PNEUMOTHORAX

A pneumothorax is defined as a collection of gas in the pleural space that results in a complete or partial collapse of the lung. A traumatic pneumothorax is caused by blunt trauma. It is usually associated with a rib fracture that causes a laceration of the lung. However, a pneumothorax can also occur from blunt trauma without a rib fracture. A spontaneous pneumothorax is common among previously healthy young adults. It usually occurs in the absence of trauma and immediately after activity, when an area of the lung tissue ruptures spontaneously. It can be caused by coughing and other simple exertions. Air can leak into the pleural space often because of the rupture of small apical blebs on the surface of the visceral pleura. There is a strong tendency towards recurrence.

As the air enters the pleural cavity from the lung with each inspiration, the air is trapped in the pleural cavity separating the lung from the chest wall. The volume of the lung is reduced from the air filling the pleural cavity. As a result, the lung can no longer expand normally. The mediastinum then shifts with deviation of the trachea toward the unaffected side because of the normal elastic recoil of the unaffected lung. If the torn or punctured side of the lung does not heal itself, the pressure will continue to build in the affected pleural cavity—causing the collapsing lung to press against the uninvolved lung and heart, compromising their efficiency. The symptoms of an athlete with a pneumothorax are a rapid progressive dyspnea, pleuritic chest pain, and shallow and rapid respirations with poor entry into the affected lung. On physical exam one can note hyperresonance to percussion of the affected area. In addition, there is a referred pain at the tip of the shoulder of the affected side. An athlete who appears cyanotic is indicative of a large pneumothorax. In addition, a weak pulse, low blood pressure, and distended neck veins are also consistent with a large pneumothorax.

Management of a pneumothorax mandates close monitoring of the vital signs. Because of the potential for a rather rapid demise, one should be prepared for possible mouth-to-mouth resuscitation. If a pneumothorax is due to a penetrating wound, an occlusive dressing should be placed to prevent additional air from entering the pleural cavity. With a pneumothorax, attempts should be made to stabilize the athlete at the playing field and transport him or her to a medical facility immediately.

At the medical facility a chest x-ray should be performed, ideally at the end of maximum expiration and in the upright position. Serial radiographs should be performed daily to assess whether there is reexpansion of the lung as free air is absorbed. If there is greater than a 30% pneumothorax, then an intercostal catheter should be placed, and the athlete should be hospitalized until the pneumothorax resolves. If a tension pneumothorax is suspected on the field, and the athlete has severe dyspnea with possible circulatory collapse, then the physician should be prepared to insert a 12- to 14-gauge needle into the pleural space at the midclavicular line between the seventh and fourth intercostal space.

After resolution of the pneumothorax one can gradually advance the athlete back to full activity over a 2- to 3-week period. It is recommended that a chest flap jacket be worn to protect this area and to prevent a reccurrence. Approximately 50% of individuals with spontaneous pneumothorax will experience a recurrence.

# RIB CONTUSION

A rib contusion is the most frequently experienced external thoracic injury in contact sports. This usually occurs from a direct blow to the chest wall involving bruising of the intercostal musculature. Clinically, the direct blow will cause the athlete to complain of pain in the area involved with the contact. If it is a severe blow, a muscle spasm may result with subsequent difficulty in breathing for a short period of time. The athlete will usually complain of an area of reproducible tenderness and sharp pain during inspiration and expiration.

The physical exam is remarkable for a palpable area of tenderness localized to a particular rib, with concomitant swelling for more severe injuries. With a contusion to the rib and surrounding area there is usually no crepitus with palpation of the rib. In addition, with a contused rib there is no pain with motion of the rib. A posterior blow to the rib cage usually results in muscular contusion rather than actual rib contusion because of the increased musculature present posteriorly. Auscultation of the lungs will reveal equal breath sounds bilaterally.

Management of a rib contusion includes application of ice and compression, and rest. In addition, pain control is an important element of the treatment because of the reproducibility of the discomfort with normal breathing. The athlete should be reassured that the persistence of the discomfort is secondary to the function of the rib musculature in normal inspiration and expiration, resulting in a prolongation of the healing process. Occasionally a complicating hematoma has to be aspirated. With a contusion to the rib cage the athlete is allowed to return to activity when he or she can tolerate the discomfort. Protective padding to the area involved is recommended. Often a chest x-ray with rib films has to be obtained to reassure the athlete that there is no underlying rib fracture.

# RIB FRACTURE

A rib fracture is usually caused by a direct blow from a blunt object or by forceful compression of the chest in one of its diameters. The complicated rib fracture is rare in a young athlete because the bones are elastic or pliable enough that they usually do not splinter into sharp pointed fragments. The concern with a splintered rib is the potential for damage to the internal mammary artery, penetration of the lung causing a pneumothorax, or penetration of the pericardium. Lower rib fractures may lacerate the liver, spleen, or kidney. Most frequently, the intercostal vessels and nerves are damaged, resulting in marked localized swelling and hematoma formation.

Clinically, the athlete will complain of significant localized pain. In addition, he or she will demonstrate persistent difficulty of breathing, suggesting a potential internal injury. The presentation of dyspnea, cyanosis, and difficulty getting enough air is indicative of decreased lung capacity. Management of this type of injury mandates immediate triage to the hospital. If the athlete's condition rapidly deteriorates, one should be prepared to aspirate the involved side to attempt to improve lung capacity. In addition, supplemental oxygen should be provided.

With an uncomplicated rib fracture the athlete will usually complain of severe localized pain accompanied by exacerbation of the pain with deep breathing, coughing, or sneezing. Muscle spasm necessitates a splinting of the chest to prevent deep breathing, lessening the amount of pain. In addition, the athlete will usually grab his or her chest, attempting to restrict motion manually.

A physical exam of an uncomplicated rib fracture is remarkable for tenderness localized directly over the rib or ribs. Pain will also be elicited in the same area with deep inspiration. In addition, a defect in the rib can be palpated with a complete fracture. Palpation may also produce crepitus. If a rib fracture is suspected, the rib should not be manipulated, so as not to further exacerbate the situation. With an uncomplicated rib fracture equal breath sounds should be audible bilaterally.

Management of an uncomplicated rib fracture entails localized treatment of the pain with ice and padding. Immobilization of the area is important to prevent motion of the rib and further injury. In this situation a local anesthetic, if injected carefully in the involved rib and surrounding ribs, is an acceptable way of decreasing the marked pain and muscle spasm.

## COSTOCHONDRAL DISLOCATION

Costochondral dislocation occurs when there is a separation of the cartilaginous anterior portion of the ribs from either the sternum medially or the body of the rib laterally. This usually occurs in contact sports. Common mechanisms are a direct blow at the junction of the rib and sternum; rib cage compression; and the arm being pulled to one side, which stretches the costochondral junction.

Clinically, the athlete usually will complain of anterior chest pain. This usually is sharp initially, and gradually it becomes stable, with intermittent pain over the site of the injury as the disrupted cartilage and the bone override each other. There may be a prominence of anterior chest pain that disappears as the cartilage clicks back into place.

Pain in the involved area is more noticeable or exacerbated by coughing or sneezing.

The physical exam is remarkable for pain on direct pressure of the area involved, pain on pressure against the corresponding rib in the axillary line, and pain on pressure downward on the sternum. With anterior displacement of the rib a palpable defect may be present. An audible click may be heard by alternating pressure on the sternum and on the involved rib or area of cartilage.

If there is no demonstrable displacement or no palpable click, one can assume that the major portion of ligamentous investiture is intact. Thus one should attempt to prevent further injury and relieve discomfort. Initial treatment of the area involves applying ice to decrease the inflammation and the swelling. An x-ray should also be obtained to rule out a rib fracture. To prevent wide excursion of the ribs and further pain, the area should be bound firmly at the lower half of the chest with the rib belt Elastoplast or an accessible strapping device. Local injection with a long-acting anesthetic is an acceptable and good means of pain control. Return to contact sports may take 6 to 8 weeks to be certain that the union after reduction is secure.

## STERNOCLAVICULAR DISLOCATION

Dislocation of the sternoclavicular joint usually occurs when an athlete falls on his or her acromioclavicular joint, and the force of the fall is transmitted medially through the clavicle to the sternoclavicular joint. Posterior dislocation of the clavicle is rare, but it is the most dangerous because there is a potential for life-threatening impingement of the great vessels, esophagus, or trachea. Anterior dislocation of the sternoclavicular joint is the most common and considered much less dangerous. In this scenario the proximal tip of the clavicle overrides the sternum.

On physical exam there is a gross displacement of the sternoclavicular joint with considerable swelling. Obviously there is disability of the upper extremity on the involved side. With posterior dislocation the athlete may present with dyspnea secondary to impingement of the trachea.

Management of sternoclavicular dislocation usually involves supporting the arm against the chest with swaths. Reduction of the sternoclavicular joint should not be attempted on the sideline. The athlete should be triaged to a medical facility for further evaluation and treatment. During this time ice should be used to minimize the pain and swelling. In addition, vital signs should be monitored carefully, especially if a posterior sternoclavicular dislocation is being considered.

# FIRST RIB FRACTURES (ISOLATED)

The first rib is short, broad, flat, and relatively thick. Though it appears to be protected low in the neck, it is an area of anatomic weakness, and injuries do occur. The first rib is attached posteriorly with the first thoracic vertebrae and anteriorly with the sternum. Thus fractures occur secondary to the following events: (1) direct external trauma; (2) indirect trauma (falling on an outstretched arm, hyperabduction of the arm, or a blow to the shoulder); and (3) fatigue or stress fractures, or violent musculature contraction.

Clinically, the athlete will complain of acute onset of pain preceded by a feeling of a snap in the shoulder. The pain may increase over several days. Pain is usually located diffusely around the clavicle or under the scapula in the shoulder. The pain is often exacerbated with movement of the shoulder, and there is the potential for weakness and paresthesias.

On physical exam one usually finds swelling and ecchymosis. In addition, one can reproduce and worsen the pain by having the athlete move his or her shoulder. The pain will be made worse, especially with abduction greater than 90 degrees. One should also assess the athlete for neurovascular impairment of the involved extremity. Potential complications of an isolated rib fracture are a rupture of the apex of the lung, pleurisy, an aortic arch aneurysm, brachial plexus syndrome, and a ruptured subclavian artery. Management involves initial application of ice and splinting the involved side. Likewise, careful and repetitive assessments of vital signs and neurovascular checks are mandatory. The athlete should be sent for an x-ray and possible angiogram if he or she is neurovascularly impaired.

# TEARS OF THE PECTORALIS MUSCLE

A tear of the pectoralis muscle usually occurs secondary to excessive muscle stress or after a direct blow to the shoulder region when the arm is in the abducted and extended position. This type of injury is extremely rare. Usually the athlete will complain of a sharp, sudden pain in the upper arm and shoulder. The athlete may report feeling a snap or a pop at the time of the injury. As stated, the arm is usually extended and in the abducted position.

The physical exam is remarkable for mild pain and weakness of flexion, adduction, and internal rotation of the affected shoulder. An area of ecchymosis and swelling in the arm and/or breast region is often evident. The injured pectoralis muscle will bulge prominently in the chest when the pectoralis major muscle contracts against resistance. With rupture of the tendon, a palpable defect may be present in the anterior axillary fold. Management usually consists of splinting the arm (to minimize movement of the involved arm) and applying ice. Conservative therapy is an acceptable form of therapy for the athlete not pursuing a sport on a collegiate or professional level. Surgical correction is recommended if the tear is complete either at the distal insertion site or the musculotendinous junction, and if the athlete is considering competing at a collegiate or professional level.

## STERNAL FRACTURES

A fracture of the sternum usually occurs through the upper portion of the sternum. The body is driven forcibly backward while the manubrium is held in place by the first and second ribs, so that the upper portion of the body overrides the lower portion. This is usually caused by either a direct blow to the sternum; violent compression force applied posteriorly (which compresses the rib cage); or hyperflexion of the trunk (which compresses the thoracic cage).

Clinically, the athlete will incur a severe blow and immediate loss of breath. He or she also will complain of persistent sternal pain that worsens with inspiration. A complete fracture of the sternum usually results in pain with normal respirations. On physical exam the athlete might have local swelling with tenderness in the immediate area of the fracture site. There also may be a possible deformity.

One of the obvious complications of a sternal fracture is flail chest with a possible pneumothorax and hemothorax. Thus while assessing the athlete with a potential sternal fracture, one should regularly reassess the breath sounds and heart sounds. Ice should be applied to the area to minimize the swelling and pain, followed by heat. Compression of the chest by a rib binder or a circumferential adhesive is advisable. Because of the aforementioned complications, the patient should be taken to the hospital for x-rays and observation overnight since damage to the underlying structures may develop insidiously over several hours.

### Bibliography

Barrett GR et al: First rib fractures in football players, *Am J Sports Med* 16:674-767, 1988.
Borrero E: Traumatic posterior displacement of the left clavicular head causing chronic extrinsic compression of the subclavian artery, *Physician Sports Med* 15:87-89, 1987.
Espinosa R et al: Acute posterior wall myocardial infarction secondary to football chest trauma, *Chest* 88:928-929, 1985.
Janda DH et al: An analysis of preventive methods for baseball-induced chest impact injuries, *Clin J Sport Med* 2:172-179, 1992.

Keating TM: Stress fracture of the sternum in a wrestler, *Am J Sports Med* 15:92-93, 1987.

Kretzler HH et al: Rupture of the pectoralis major muscle, *Am J Sports Med* 17:453-458, 1989.

Kulund D: *The injured athlete*, Philadelphia, 1988, JB Lippincott.

McEntire JE et al: Rupture of the pectoralis major muscle. *J Bone Joint Surg* 54A:1040-1045, 1972.

O'Donoghue DH: *Treatment of injuries to athletes*, Philadelphia, 1984, WB Saunders.

Pfeiffer RP et al: Case report: spontaneous pneumothorax in a jogger, *Physician Sports Med* 8:65-67, 1980.

Phillips EH et al: First rib fractures: incidence of vascular injury and indications for angiography, *Surgery* 89:42-47, 1981.

Reut RC et al: Pectoralis major rupture, *Physician Sports Med* 19:89-96, 1991.

Viano DC et al: Fatal chest injury by baseball impact in children: a brief review, *Clin J Sport Med* 2:161-165, 1992.

Viano DC et al: Mechanism of fatal chest injury by baseball impact: development of an experimental model, *Clin J Sport Med* 2:166-171, 1992.

Yee ES: Isolated first rib fracture: clinical significance after blunt chest trauma, *Ann Thorac Surg* 32:278-282, 1981.

## Chapter 6

# Abdominal and genital injuries

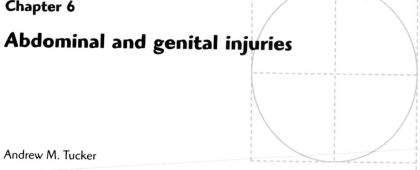

Andrew M. Tucker

Abdominal injuries in sports cover a broad spectrum, from minor contusions and strains to life-threatening emergencies. Sports medicine providers who care for athletes in contact and collision sports must be systematic in the evaluation of these injuries and aware of the pitfalls associated with the diagnostic process. The clinician must feel comfortable with the basics of emergency medical treatment in the event of a catastrophic injury.

The purpose of this chapter is to review the mechanism of abdominal injury, as well as to review on-field and training room diagnostic considerations and initial treatment. Return-to-play criteria are discussed. A section on genitourinary injuries is also included.

## ABDOMINAL INJURIES

### MECHANISM OF INJURY

Abdominal trauma may be categorized as penetrating or blunt trauma. Most sports-related abdominal injuries are caused by blunt trauma through an intact abdominal wall.[8] The muscle and aponeurotic structures provide some protection for the abdominal organs. In addition, the inferior aspect of the rib cage helps protect the liver, spleen, and kidneys. It should be remembered that injury to the lower rib structures may result in secondary injury to underlying organs (Fig. 6-1). With the exception of some positions in team sports (e.g., hockey goalie, baseball catcher), many sports uniforms do not include significant abdominal or flank protection.

Blunt trauma through an intact abdominal wall may result from an object (e.g., a baseball) striking the athlete or from a moving athlete striking another participant or a stationary object (e.g., a goal post, a bench, or the ground). The solid organs (e.g., the kidneys and liver) are more

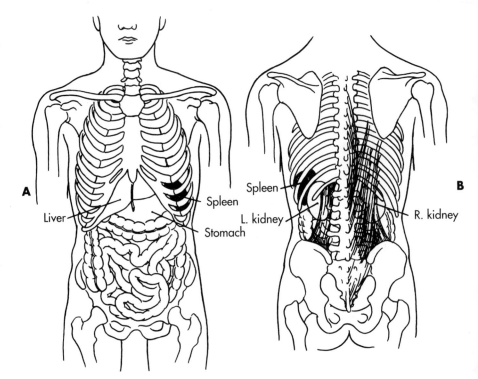

**Fig. 6-1.** Anatomic relationships of abdominal organs. **A,** Anterior view. **B,** Posterior view. (From Olsen WR: Abdominal trauma in the athlete. In Schneider RC et al, editors: *Sports injuries: mechanisms, prevention, and treatment,* Baltimore, 1985, Williams & Wilkins. Reproduced by permission.)

vulnerable to injury from blunt trauma.[8] A hollow viscus may be ruptured with a "blow out" type of injury in which blunt trauma results in a significant increase in luminal pressure.[8] Severe deceleration can be an important mechanism in abdominal injury.[4] Abdominal viscera that are tethered or attached to the abdominal wall are prone to injury from severe deceleration forces, which may cause a laceration of the viscera or disruption of the vascular pedicle to an organ.[4]

The muscles of the abdominal wall may be strained or contused from blunt trauma, causing significant disability to the athlete.

## CLINICAL DIAGNOSIS

The clinical assessment of abdominal injuries is often difficult. An athlete sustaining a serious intraabdominal injury initially may have mild symp-

**Table 6**
**PHYSICAL EXAMINATION OF THE ABDOMEN AFTER BLUNT TRAUMA FREQUENTLY IS MISLEADING**

| Signs of visceral injury on initial abdominal examination | Percent of patients | Incidence of significant intraabdominal injury (%) |
| --- | --- | --- |
| Obvious | 22 | 80 |
| Equivocal | 46 | 35 |
| Negative | 12 | 43 |
| Unreliable because of head or spine injury | 19 | 35 |

From Olsen WR: Abdominal trauma in the athlete. In Schneider RC et al, editors: *Sports injuries: mechanisms, prevention, and treatment,* Baltimore, 1985, Williams & Wilkins. Reproduced by permission.

tomatology. On the contrary, severe abdominal wall contusions or muscular strains can be quite disabling to the athlete. One author has documented that the initial abdominal examination may not be a reliable guide to the severity of intraabdominal injury (Table 6).[8]

The evaluation must be performed quickly to minimize time to hospital care in those rare cases of emergency abdominal trauma. When there is uncertainty about the severity of the trauma, frequent serial evaluations are performed to detect subtle trends or changes in the patient's condition.

The history begins with a thorough understanding of the mechanism of injury. A description of blunt trauma should prompt a short differential diagnosis based on the underlying anatomy. The history also includes the location of pain, though this is often vague and diffuse after abdominal injury. Radiation of pain may be significant, given that pathology under the right or left diaphragm may be referred to the right and left shoulder areas, respectively.[5]

Nausea is common after a blow to the abdomen, with progressive nausea and vomiting of greater significance. If there is rapid bleeding, symptoms of shock and hypovolemia (such as postural dizziness) may be present. Respiratory symptoms may indicate a significant diaphragmatic injury with associated chest pathology.

A systematic physical examination follows the brief history. For the most severely injured patient, rapid assessment of vital signs is necessary. The abdomen and flank should be exposed for examination. Inspection may find contusion, abrasion, or abdominal distention. Auscultation of the abdomen may be helpful. Absence of bowel sounds may indicate a significant injury. However, the presence of bowel sounds does not exclude a serious intraabdominal injury.[5]

Light and deep palpation is performed to elicit areas of tenderness or masses from enlarged organs. Tenderness may be focal or diffuse. The examiner should note areas of spasm or guarding and signs of peritoneal irritation including rebound tenderness. Subcutaneous emphysema may be palpable in cases of rib injuries with disruption of the pleural cavity. The examiner should remember to briefly examine the chest for areas of tenderness or deformity and auscultation of the heart and lungs.

In cases in which the athlete is taken from the playing field to the training room, a rectal exam and stool guaiac test may be indicated to evaluate for gastrointestinal tract bleeding. If genitourinary tract pathology is suspected, a dipstick urine test can be used to evaluate for hematuria.[3]

## DIFFERENTIAL DIAGNOSIS

While the clinician should recognize that any of the intraabdominal organs may be injured, the immediate priority is determining whether a life-threatening injury exists, rather than identifying the specific organ or structures involved. Most simply, the differential diagnosis includes an abdominal wall injury (strain, contusion, hematoma) versus a more significant intraabdominal injury.

Therefore a valuable approach to the differential diagnosis would be to consider the acuteness of the situation. An athlete who has signs and symptoms of vascular instability should be presumed to have suffered a significant laceration or disruption of an intraabdominal organ. Symptoms and signs that evolve from an apparently stable situation to one of increasing pain, nausea, and vomiting (and possible vascular instability) may represent slow bleeding of a solid organ or a laceration of a hollow organ such as the small or large intestine.[5] One case report describes a jejunal rupture in a football player who had already returned to the game before symptoms worsened.[6] An exception to the subacute presentation of a disrupted hollow organ may involve a disruption of the stomach, in which spillage of the extremely acidic stomach contents can present in a more acute fashion.[5]

Stable and slowly improving symptoms make an isolated abdominal wall injury more likely, although the clinician must never forget the possibility of an associated intraabdominal injury.

## ON-FIELD TREATMENT

As the most likely life-threatening complication from blunt abdominal trauma is rapid bleeding, the clinician must minimize the time necessary to transport the player to definitive hospital care. Thus the clinician's highest priority is to determine if a life-threatening injury has occurred.

In an emergency situation the health care provider must activate the emergency medical system and prepare the player for rapid ambulance transport to the nearest trauma facility. All sports medicine providers should be certified in basic life support.

Basic life support includes a rapid primary survey of adequacy of airway, presence of respirations, and assessment of the circulatory status.[7] The secondary survey would include a brief neurologic assessment and basic care of any obvious fractures or external bleeding. The clinician may be called upon to start an intravenous line and to coordinate moving the player to the emergency vehicle for transport to the hospital.

Physicians covering contact and collision sports should have access to basic equipment that allows them to accomplish the aforementioned services. This includes equipment for airway management (oral airways, resuscitation, and intubation equipment), a stethoscope and sphygmomanometer, intravenous supplies, and possibly cardiac monitoring equipment. Sterile dressings for wound management and splints for fractures and/or dislocations should also be available.[5]

In the hospital, initial evaluation includes a complete blood count, type, and cross-match; serum amylase; coagulation profile; and chemistries.[8] Plain films of the abdomen and chest evaluate for free air or evidence of obstruction. When signs of rapid bleeding are evident, trauma surgeons often use peritoneal lavage to determine the presence of intraabdominal bleeding.[8] Other tests used in the acute setting include computed tomography (CT) with contrast and ultrasound.[8]

Injuries that do not show evidence of cardiovascular compromise but are judged by the clinician to be potentially serious pose difficult decisions. In these situations, the clinician may withhold the athlete from further play and closely observe him or her with frequent examinations to determine any changes or trends in the player's condition. Transport to a hospital for further evaluation would be indicated for worsening abdominal pain or nausea and vomiting, or the earliest signs of change in cardiovascular status. However, if signs and symptoms stabilize or slowly improve, then transport may not be necessary. For persistent symptoms, noninvasive tests such as ultrasound or CT with contrast are sometimes used to help confirm the absence of significant intraabdominal trauma. Many would err on the side of caution and order such tests since the consequences of missing a subacute injury to the abdomen could be significant.

If the clinician judges the injury to involve the abdominal wall only, then a decision must be made regarding return to play. Considerations include the level of pain and limitations in strength and motion, the adequacy of padding and protection of the affected area, and the ability of the athlete to withstand further trauma to the injured area. Ice may be used on the sideline to help minimize the acute pain reaction.

## RETURN-TO-PLAY CRITERIA

Return to play following abdominal wall injuries will depend on resolution of pain and tenderness, and restoration of normal range of motion and abdominal strength (with the possibility of using protective padding to hasten the return).

Little has been written about the return to play following more severe intraabdominal injuries. For contusions to the solid organs such as the kidneys, spleen, and liver, one author recommends a 2- to 3-week period of rest.[7] Guidelines for return to training and competition are lacking, and one can presume these decisions must be individualized, depending on the clinical situation and sport.

For severe intraabdominal injuries that result in lacerations, significant bleeding, and surgery, any decision about a return to sports must be individualized, and the decision should be made in conjunction with the player's surgeon. One author recommends that severe wounds to the liver preclude return to contact or collision sports secondary to scarring in the liver and the possibility of recurrent injury.[8] In one case history of an athlete who suffered a duodenal hematoma, the player was hospitalized for 4 days. Surgery was not required, but the player was withheld from football for the rest of the season. How much time remained in the season is unknown; however, the author does indicate that the player returned to competitive basketball and baseball immediately following that football season. No complications were reported.[4]

One practical question is the consideration of return to play following abdominal surgery, with respect to strength of the postoperative wound. Guidelines have been provided for return to activity following specific surgeries (Table 7).[8]

A common scenario confronting a physician concerns the return of an athlete to sports following mononucleosis. It is well known that splenic enlargement accompanies a significant percentage of patients with mononucleosis.[3] The reported incidence of splenic rupture in patients with mononucleosis is 0.1% to 0.2%.[3] There is disagreement about when to allow return to activity after acute mononucleosis. One author offers that noncontact sports are to be avoided for a full 4 months, and contact sports are to be avoided for 6 months.[8] Other authors are less conservative. One source indicates that it is prudent to wait for 3 weeks to start training and 4 weeks for strenuous activities, assuming splenic enlargement is absent. The same author recommends ultrasound of the spleen if there is concern about persistent enlargement.[3] A similar recommendation from

**Table 7**
**RECOMMENDED TIME (IN WEEKS) BEFORE ALLOWING THE HEALTHY ATHLETE TO RETURN TO ACTIVITY AFTER AN ABDOMINAL OPERATION**

| | Return to classes | Supervised progressive exercise and conditioning | Noncontact sports | All activities including contact sports |
|---|---|---|---|---|
| Indirect hernias in children | 1 | 2 | 3 | 4 |
| Small indirect hernias in teenagers or adults | 1 | 3 | 4 | 6 |
| Appendectomy (McBurney incision) | 1 | 3 | 4 | 6 |
| Other uncomplicated abdominal operations | 2 | 4 | 8 | 12 |

From Olsen WR: Abdominal trauma in the athlete. In Schneider RC et al, editors: *Sports injuries: mechanisms, prevention, and treatment,* Baltimore, 1985, Williams & Wilkins. Reproduced by permission.

another source indicates that return to full activity can begin in 1 month if the patient feels able and if the spleen is of normal size.[1,2] The general consensus of sports medicine practitioners would seem to follow the latter two opinions.

## GENITAL INJURIES

Genitourinary injuries are uncommon in sports but may occur in any high velocity activity or contact-collision sport. The kidney, perhaps the most commonly injured genitourinary organ, is considered in previous sections of this chapter.

The ureter is well protected in its retroperitoneal position but may sustain contusions, hematomas, or lacerations, usually in association with other intraabdominal injuries.[7] Abdominal pain from ureteral injury may be minimal, and intravenous pyelogram (IVP) is the primary diagnostic tool.[7] Lacerations require surgical repair.[5]

The bladder may be contused or ruptured. A ruptured bladder is more likely to occur when the bladder is full.[7] A contusion of the bladder would present with microscopic or gross hematuria and possibly localized tenderness over the bladder. A ruptured bladder with extravasation of urine would cause increasing pain and abdominal tenderness.[7] Bladder injuries are best diagnosed by IVP or cystography.[5] A ruptured bladder requires surgical treatment; a contused bladder can generally be managed by the insertion of a Foley catheter and with observation.[5]

Urethral injuries in the male can be divided into anterior injuries (portion distal to the fixed triangular ligament) and posterior injuries (located within the triangular ligament and the prostatic urethra).[5] Posterior urethral injuries are usually secondary to pelvic fractures.[5] Mild to moderate trauma of the anterior urethra may cause hemorrhage and possible obstruction secondary to clots, whereas severe injuries may cause urethral disruption with extravasation of urine.[5] Tests may include urethrography or endoscopy.

Contusions to the scrotum can usually be treated with cold packs and elevation. Surgical exploration may be necessary for evacuation of hematoma or repair of testicular laceration.[7]

Urethral injuries in the female are rare, but they may occur from blunt trauma during sports such as gymnastics or cycling and involve laceration or contusion to the distal urethra.[5]

External genitalia injuries in females may occur in gymnastics or various jumping sports such as pole vault. These injuries generally can be treated with cold packs and bed rest. For significant injuries, a gynecologic consult is indicated.[7]

# References

1. Committee on Sports Medicine and Fitness of the American Academy of Pediatrics, Sports Medicine: *Health care for young athletes*, ed 2, Elk Grove Village, Ill, 1991, The Academy.
2. Eichner ER: Infectious mononucleosis: recognition and management in athletes, *Physician Sports Med* 15:61-70, 1987.
3. Green GA: Gastrointestinal disorders in the athlete, *Clin Sports Med* 11:453-470, 1992.
4. Henderson JM, Puffer JC: Abdominal pain in a football player: a case conference, *Physician Sports Med* 17:47-52, 1989.
5. Moncure AC, Wilken EW Jr: Injuries involving the abdomen, viscera and genitourinary system. In Vinger PF, Hoerner EF, editors: *Sports injuries: the unthwarted epidemic*, Littleton, Mass, 1986, PSG.
6. Murphy CP, Drez D Jr: Jejunal rupture in a football player, *Am J Sports Med* 15:184-185, 1987.
7. Mustalish AC, Quash ET: Sports injuries to the chest and abdomen. In Scott WN, Misonson B, Nicholas JA, editors: *Principles of sports medicine*, Baltimore, 1984, Williams & Wilkins.
8. Olsen WR: Abdominal trauma in the athlete. In Schneider RC et al, editor: *Sports injuries: mechanisms, prevention, and treatment*, Baltimore, 1985, Williams & Wilkins.

# Chapter 7

# Heat problems and dehydration

Debra S. Williams

Heat illnesses are associated with a variety of athletic activities, including preseason football endurance races, soccer, and field hockey, as well as various types of summer sports camps. The spectrum of these conditions can range from benign to fatal. Athletes participating in high temperature and high humidity environments are increasingly susceptible to heat-related problems. Increased knowledge and preventive measures have decreased the incidence of heat-related illness, but there must continue to be awareness, recognition, and appropriate treatment for these conditions.

## BASIC PHYSIOLOGY

Major factors involved in heat intolerance are the body's heat production during exercise combined with the effect of the environmental temperature and humidity. The body's response to its heat production and the environment creates a balance in which heat production equals heat loss. Hypothalamic neural control is the center of the body's effort to withstand endogenous and exogenous heat challenges.

Heat production is proportional to body weight. Heat loss is proportional to body surface area. For each 1° C rise in core body temperature, metabolic demands for oxygen consumption increase by 6% to 7% of normal.

To prevent excessive rise in core body temperature, there is increased blood flow to the skin and increased sweating. Heat dissipation is primarily by evaporation. During exercise 80% of total heat removed is by sweat evaporation.

For a 70-kg adult male, sweat production is approximately 1 L per hour of exercise. For every 100 ml of sweat evaporated, there is a 1° C decrease in the rise of the mean core body temperature.

Muscle demands increase, thereby requiring increased cardiac output during heavy exercise. Mechanisms to increase heat loss include cutaneous vasodilatation, sweating, and increased respiratory rate. The immediate response is vasodilatation of the skin vessels, which—with increased blood flow to the skin and increased sweat production—maximizes losses through radiation and convection. With moderate heat exposure the increased blood flow to the skin is achieved at the expense of flow to other organs. Greater heat stress increases pulse pressure to maintain cardiac output. The body can reach a critical point at which a higher heart rate cannot be maintained.

## ENVIRONMENTAL EFFECTS

High levels of heat and humidity severely limit the exercising body's ability to dissipate heat. Coaches, athletes, trainers, and physicians cannot depend only on how "hot or humid" it feels to judge heat stress. More objective measurements are necessary to make appropriate adjustments in exercise duration and intensity.

Weather reports can provide approximate temperature and humidity readings, and relative degrees of heat stress can be determined using a heat stress chart.

A sling psychrometer is used to measure dry bulb (DB) and wet bulb (WB) temperatures at the activity site. Relative humidity is then determined from a chart provided with the instrument.

The heat index thermometer is a more complex and expensive system used to measure WB, DB, and black bulb (BB) temperatures. It provides a measure of the radiant heat gained in the heat stress index. The wet bulb global temperature (WBGT) index is compared with published guidelines that indicate relative levels of heat-stress risk.

## HEAT ILLNESSES

### HEAT SYNCOPE

Heat syncope occurs when an athlete stands still after vigorous exercise. There is maximal vasodilatation of peripheral blood vessels with resultant venous pooling. This venous pooling causes decreased cardiac output and stroke volume accompanied either by the clinical symptoms of severe light-headedness and dizziness, or by a transient fainting episode. The core body temperature remains normal. Treatment consists of placing the athlete in the prone position with legs elevated in a cool shaded area. Oral fluids may help alleviate symptoms but are not required unless there was a hypohydrated state before the syncopal episode. Recovery is usually rapid after brief recumbency, and the athlete may return to mild activity with increase to full participation as tolerated.

## HEAT CRAMPS

Heat cramps usually involve extremely painful contractions of the large muscle groups of the legs but may also involve abdominal and intracostal muscles, mimicking an acute condition in the abdomen. The cramps are due to decreased hydration and a lack of balance between salt and water in the muscles. The cramps usually do not respond to massaging the muscle. Treatment consists of rest from exertional activity and passive stretching. Fluid replacement with ingestion of water or hypotonic saline solution is necessary. For more rapid results, administration of 1 to 2 L of half-normal saline solution may be considered. Activity may be resumed when hydration and electrolyte balance are normal.

Heat cramps may be recurrent if cumulative deficits of fluid and electrolytes exist. Prevention includes adequate hydration before and throughout exercise.

## HEAT EXHAUSTION

Heat exhaustion is a more severe heat syndrome, and it is the most common form of heat intolerance in athletes. There are two types of heat exhaustion: water depletion, which is the most common; or salt depletion, which is less common. The syndrome is characterized by severe fatigue, profound weakness and sweating, nausea, and diarrhea. Mental status is usually normal to slightly impaired. Treatment consists of lying down in a cool area and fluid replacement until normal body weight is obtained and polyuria begins. The most important oral fluid is water, although controversy remains about whether the addition of glucose helps or hurts. The athlete may or may not need intravenous (IV) fluids. If cooling and oral fluids fail to provide clinical improvement, administration of a liter of IV fluids should be started while obtaining electrolytes. The athlete should not be allowed to return to vigorous activity until normal body weight is reached, and, in severe cases, until normal electrolytes are restored.

## HEAT STROKE

Heat stroke is a *medical emergency* characterized by extreme hyperthermia, failure of the body's thermoregulatory mechanism, and profound central nervous system dysfunction. Because there may be permanent nerve damage secondary to hyperpyrexia, rapid and vigorous treatment is essential for full recovery. The absence of sweating and presence of moderate dehydration in the exercising athlete intensify hyperpyrexia. For every 1° F rise in core body temperature, metabolism increases 7%, creating a vicious cycle. With fluid loss from exercise, the heat regulatory system fails, and the central sweating mechanism stops to avoid further dehydration. As the heat generated by metabolic activity builds up, body temperature rises, but the skin stays dry. Because heat illness is cumulative, heat stroke usually occurs when the ambient temperature is 95° F for 2 days or longer and when the relative humidity is in the range of 50% to 75%. This condition has a 50% to 75% fatality rate, with 80% of fatalities being due to circulatory failure.

The key to diagnosis is a rectal temperature of 105° F or greater. Warning symptoms are aggressiveness, irritability, emotional instability, and hysteria; progressing to apathy, failure to answer questions, and disorientation. The athlete may have an unsteady gait and a glassy stare. Hot, dry skin accompanies the final signs of collapse and unconsciousness. Initially, the pulse is rapid and full. As the changes become established and tissue is damaged by body heat, vasomotor collapse occurs; blood pressure falls; and the pulse is rapid and weak. Heat stroke progresses rapidly to cardiovascular and central nervous system collapse. There are a myriad of electrolyte and metabolic imbalances that require careful monitoring.

Treatment must be initiated as soon as a diagnosis is made. The ambulance should be called immediately. While awaiting emergency transportation, the athlete's clothing should be removed and he or she should be immersed in a cool-water bath. Alternately, cover the athlete's body with wet sheets and compresses, and have a fan blowing over the body. External cooling may be stopped when rectal temperature reaches 102° F. Many heat stroke patients require airway management, oxygenation, cautious rehydration to avoid cerebral edema, and circulatory support with intensive-care cardiac and metabolic monitoring.

## PREVENTING HEAT ILLNESS

Acclimatization is the body's adaptation to heat stress and increased capacity to work in high environmental temperature and humidity. Depending on the physical demands of the sport, acclimatization may take from 7 days to several weeks. The preparation should be gradual and begin with initial workouts of 30 to 45 minutes, increasing to 2 hours. Acclimatization results in a lower resting body temperature, lessened increase in pulse and respiratory rate, and earlier sweating. These modifications in cardiovascular, neural, and hormonal physiology result in reduced risk of patient suffering from heat illness.

During hot, humid weather, practices should be held in the early morning or late afternoon to avoid the most intense heat. Early in the season, night games should be scheduled when possible. Equipment and uniforms should be light-weight, porous, and light in color. Sleeves should be short, and socks should be low. Perspiration-soaked uniforms should be changed during practice to increase cooling by evaporation. As much skin as possible should be exposed to air.

Hydration is the key to preventing heat illness. Free intake of fluids during practice sessions and games should be encouraged. In extremes of heat and humidity, regular fluid breaks should be scheduled no less than every half hour. A rule of thumb for water replacement should be 1 pt for each pound lost, or 10 oz every 30 minutes. Thirst is an inadequate gauge for determining fluid loss. Only approximately 50% of body fluid loss is made up in response to thirst. Electrolyte replacement is usually unnecessary for individuals with a normal diet, unless an event lasts more than 1 hour. Commercially available sports drinks may be used if the glucose concentration does not exceed 5% to 8%. It is still recommended that they be diluted at least twofold. Drinks containing over 10% glucose will usually cause stomach cramps, nausea, diarrhea, and decreased gastric emptying during exercise. Soft drinks and fruit juices fall into that category. Fructose is absorbed more slowly and is also more likely to cause gastrointestinal distress. Sports drinks may be beneficial to help replace glycogen stores for exercise lasting longer than 60 to 90 minutes.

To counteract the risk of cumulative hypohydration, all athletes involved in vigorous exercise should be weighed nude before and after each practice session. Those with body weight loss of 2% will begin to have some impairment of their thermoregulatory ability. A 3% loss or greater causes deterioration of performance parameters. A 4% to 5% loss shows decreases of 20% to 30% of muscular work. No player should be allowed to return to play until fluid loss is replaced and normal weight achieved.

All personnel involved with athletics should have a clear understanding of heat illness, its causes, and its treatment. Medical personnel should be able to give sound advice on prevention, recognition, and treatment of heat illness. Good communication among coaches, athletes, and training staffs is imperative. Emphasis should be placed on environmental factors, acclimatization, clothing, and fluid replacement. The old adage "An ounce of prevention is worth a pound of cure" is more than true in the case of heat illness.

## Bibliography

Bracker MD: Environmental and thermal injury, *Clin Sports Med* 11:419-436, 1992.

Coleman E: Sports science exchange, *Sports Drink Update* 1:190-194, 1988.

Environmental problems. In Hunter-Griffin LY, editor: *Athletic training and sports medicine*, Rosemont, IL, 1991, American Academy of Orthopaedic Surgeons.

Guyton AC: *Human physiology and mechanisms of disease*, Philadelphia, 1982, WB Saunders.

Mellion MB, Shelton G, Grandjean A: *Office management of sports injuries and athletic problems*, St Louis, 1988, Mosby–Year Book.

Millard-Stafford M: Fluid replacement during exercise in the heat, *Sports Med* 13:223-233, 1992.

Murphy RJ: Heat illness in the athlete, *Am J Sports Med* 12:258-261, 1984.

Peterson L, Renstrom P: *Sports injuries, their prevention and treatment*, St Louis, 1986, Mosby–Year Book.

Roberts WO: Managing heatstroke, *Physician Sports Med* 20:17-28, 1992.

Scott J: Heat related illness, *Postgrad Med* 85:154-164, June 1989.

Stanitski CL: Environmental stress. In DeLee JC, Drez D, editors: *Orthopaedic sports medicine*, vol 2, Philadelphia, 1994, WB Saunders.

Sutton JR: Environmental effects and their control. In Ryan AJ, Allman FL Jr, editors: *Sports medicine*, San Diego, 1989, Academic Press.

# Chapter 8

# Brachial plexus injuries

Alan G. Posta, Jr.
William G. Clancy, Jr.
Emory J. Alexander

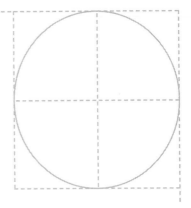

A wide spectrum of head and neck injuries may occur in the athlete. Brachial plexus injuries are uncommon in sports other than American football. Hirasawa and Sakakida reported only 66 among 1167 (5.7%) cases of sports-related peripheral nerve and brachial plexus injuries over an 18-year period.[30] They noted that Takazawa treated 28 peripheral nerve injuries among 9550 sports injuries over a 5-year period at the Japanese Athletic Association clinic.[54] Clarke, however, reported a brachial plexus injury incidence of 2.2 injuries per 100 players per year among United States high school and college football players over a 4-year period.[14] Clancy and colleagues reported a 30% to 50% incidence of transitory brachial plexus injuries over the course of a high school or college career.[13]

The brachial plexus is a complex neural structure that originates with cervical and thoracic nerve roots and reorganizes the sensory and motor contributions into peripheral nerves. Because of its location, the brachial plexus is susceptible to blunt and penetrating trauma, traction, compression, and inflammatory conditions. During athletic competition the brachial plexus may be injured in a variety of ways. The extent of these seemingly minimal injuries may not be fully appreciated by the player, coach, trainer, therapist, and physician. The appropriate treatment and ultimate outcome depend on the location of the lesion, the mechanism of injury, and the severity of injury. Prompt recognition, appropriate assessment, and proper treatment are essential for the safe and timely return of the injured athlete to participation.

## ANATOMY

An understanding of the anatomy of the brachial plexus is essential for establishing an accurate diagnosis and prognosis in brachial plexus

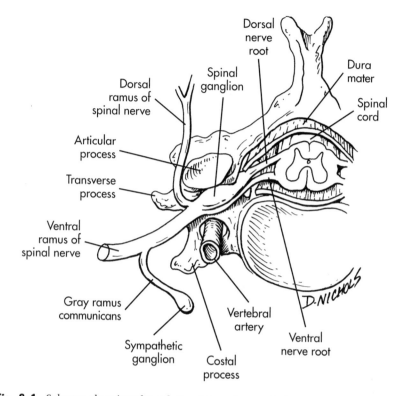

**Fig. 8-1.** Scheme showing the relationships of a cervical nerve and its ganglion to a cervical vertebra. (Redrawn from Williams PL, Warwick R, Dyson M, Bannister LH: *Gray's anatomy,* ed 37, Edinburgh, 1989, Churchill Livingstone.)

injuries. Spinal nerves from cervical root levels five through eight and the first thoracic root contribute to the brachial plexus. A prefixed plexus is defined as a brachial plexus with a substantial contribution from C4, whereas a postfixed plexus receives a significant contribution from T2.[34]

The spinal nerves that form the brachial plexus contain motor, sensory, and sympathetic fibers. The motor fibers exit the spinal cord via the ventral (anterior) root, and the sensory fibers exit via the dorsal (posterior) root. These roots combine at each level near or within the intervertebral foramen to form the nerve roots (Fig. 8-1). The sympathetic fibers join the spinal nerves via the rami communicantes.

The motor and sensory axons have ganglia that contain cell bodies for the nerves. The motor ganglia or anterior horn cells are located within the spinal cord. The cell bodies of the sensory nerves in the dorsal root are located within the dorsal root ganglia, situated just proximal to the confluence of the ventral and dorsal roots in the region of the intervertebral foramen outside the spinal cord. The spinal nerves divide into anterior and posterior primary rami after exiting from the intervertebral foramen. The posterior primary rami innervate the posterior paraspinal skin and musculature of the neck and trunk. The anterior primary rami coalesce to form the brachial plexus and lie between the anterior and middle scalene muscles.

A preganglionic brachial plexus injury, such as a root avulsion, is defined as a lesion that occurs proximal to the dorsal root ganglia. In this type of injury both the ventral and dorsal roots are injured. The motor component will undergo Wallerian degeneration, and denervation will be present in the distribution of both the anterior and posterior primary rami. The sensory neuron will remain in continuity with the afferent nerve, but sensation is absent because of the disruption of the connection between the dorsal root ganglia and the spinal cord. A postganglionic lesion occurs distal to the dorsal root ganglion. Sensory neurons will no longer remain in continuity with the afferent nerve. Denervation of muscles innervated by the anterior primary rami occurs. The paraspinal muscles of the neck and trunk are spared because the posterior primary rami are unaffected. A preganglionic root avulsion type of injury has a poor prognosis, whereas postganglionic lesions may demonstrate the potential for spontaneous recovery or recovery secondary to surgical repair or reconstruction, depending on the severity of the injury.

The ventral primary rami unite just proximal to the clavicle to form three trunks: upper (C5 to C6), middle (C7), and lower (C8 to T1) (Fig. 8-2). The site of confluence of C5 and C6 is known as Erb's point. Between the take off of the dorsal rami and Erb's point, C5 contributes a branch to the phrenic nerve (diaphragm); the long thoracic nerve (serratus anterior) arises from C5 through C7; and the dorsal scapular nerve (rhomboids) arises from C5. The suprascapular nerve (supraspinatus, infraspinatus) and nerve to the subclavius (subclavius) arise distal to Erb's point from the upper trunk. Postganglionic injuries of C5 to C6 proximal to Erb's point represent a peripheral nerve injury with loss of serratus anterior, rhomboid, and C5 to C6 function. This distinguishes nerve root injuries from upper trunk injuries that do not affect long thoracic or dorsal scapular nerve functions.

The primary trunks divide below the clavicle into the anterior and posterior divisions. Each division contributes to the formation of three cords that are named according to their relationship to the axillary artery. The three posterior divisions combine to form the posterior cord. The posterior cord (C5 to T1) has three branches: the upper subscapular nerve (subscapularis), the lower subscapular nerve (subscapularis, teres major), and the thoracodorsal nerve (latissimus dorsi). The axillary and radial nerves are the terminal branches of the posterior cord. The lateral cord (C5 to C7) is formed from the anterior division of the upper and middle

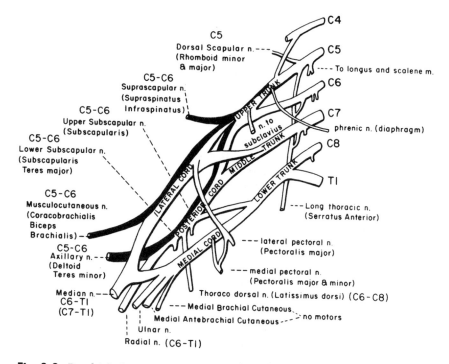

**Fig. 8-2.** Brachial plexus. (From Clancy WG Jr, Brand RL, Bergfield JA: Upper trunk brachial plexus injuries in contact sports, *Am J Sports Med* 5:209-216, 1977.)

trunks. The lateral cord gives rise to the lateral pectoral nerve (pectoralis major). The lateral cord then divides into the musculocutaneous nerve and the lateral portion of the median nerve. The medial cord (C8 through T1) is derived from the anterior division of the lower trunk. The medial pectoral nerve (pectoralis major, pectoralis minor) arises from the medial cord. The medial brachial cutaneous nerve and the medial antebrachial cutaneous nerve are two sensory branches off the medial cord. The medial cord terminates by dividing into the ulnar nerve and the medial portion of the median nerve (Table 8).

## CLASSIFICATION OF NERVE INJURIES

Seddon classified peripheral nerve injuries into three types: neurapraxia, axonotmesis, and neurotmesis.[48] This classification was designed to correlate histologic and clinical findings with prognosis. Any significant brachial plexus injury may result in variable amounts of damage to indi-

**Table 8**
**MAJOR BRANCHES OF THE BRACHIAL PLEXUS**

| Peripheral nerve | Root composition | Origin |
|---|---|---|
| Phrenic | C5 | Cervical root |
| Long thoracic | C5, C6, C7 | Cervical roots |
| Dorsal scapular | C5 | Cervical root |
| Suprascapular | C5, C6 | Upper trunk |
| Subclavius | C5, C6 | Upper trunk |
| Upper subscapular | C5 | Posterior cord |
| Lower subscapular | C5, C6 | Posterior cord |
| Thoracodorsal | C7, C8 | Posterior cord |
| Lateral pectoral | C5, C6, C7 | Lateral cord |
| Medial pectoral | C8, T1 | Medial cord |
| Medial brachial cutaneous | C8, T1 | Medial cord |
| Medial antebrachial cutaneous | C8, T1 | Medial cord |
| Axillary | C5, C6 | Posterior cord |
| Radial | C6, C7, C8 | Posterior cord |
| Musculocutaneous | C5, C6 | Lateral cord |
| Median | C5, C6, C7, C8, T1 | Medial and lateral cords |
| Ulnar | C8, T1 | Medial cord |

Modified with permission from Hershman EB: Brachial plexus injuries, *Clin Sports Med* 9:311-329, 1990.

vidual neural fibers within a given nerve, resulting in a spectrum of symptoms including neurapraxia, axonotmesis, and neurotmesis.

Neurapraxia is the mildest lesion and represents a minor contusion or compression of a peripheral nerve, resulting in edema or localized demyelinization of the axon sheath without intrinsic axonal destruction.[15-17] Transmission of impulses is physiologically interrupted at the site of injury. Neuronal function returns from within minutes up to 3 weeks postinjury when remyelinization is complete. Neurophysiologic studies are normal at that time.

Axonotmesis represents a more significant injury, resulting in axonal disruption without significant injury to the supporting stroma including the endoneurium, perineurium, and epineurium (Fig. 8-3). The entire distal axon will undergo Wallerian degeneration, and complete regeneration must occur for functional recovery. Because the neural tubes remain intact, regeneration can occur. Electromyographic (EMG) studies at 3

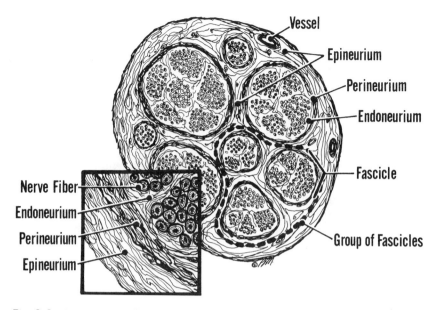

Vessel

Epineurium

Perineurium

Endoneurium

Fascicle

Nerve Fiber

Endoneurium

Perineurium

Epineurium

Group of Fascicles

**Fig. 8-3.** Cross-sectional anatomy of a peripheral nerve. (Illustration by Elizabeth Roselius, copyright © 1993. Reprinted with permission from Wilgis EFS, Brushart TM: Nerve repair and grafting. In Green DP, editor: *Operative hand surgery,* ed 3, New York, 1993, Churchill Livingstone.)

weeks postinjury reveal fibrillation and positive sharp waves, with loss of motor unit potentials in muscles innervated by damaged nerves. Overall recovery is dependent on the quality of axonal regeneration and reinnervation of the denervated muscles and sensory receptors. Following recovery, EMG studies may demonstrate large motor unit potentials.

Neurotmesis is the most severe level of injury, with complete anatomic severance of the nerve or extensive avulsion or crushing of the nerve such that the endoneurium and supporting stroma are disrupted. Significant spontaneous recovery or complete recovery following surgical repair or reconstruction is unlikely because of the disruption of the neural tube. EMG studies will demonstrate acute (3 weeks) and subsequently chronic (1 year) denervation patterns.

Sunderland has more recently provided criteria for classification of nerve injuries.[52,53] A Sunderland first degree injury corresponds to a Seddon grade 1 or neurapraxic lesion in which there is a block to nerve conduction without morphologic changes in the nerve. No Wallerian degeneration occurs, and full clinical recovery can be expected within 2 to 4 weeks. Loss of motor function and sensory deficits are transitory.

A Sunderland second degree injury is equivalent to a Seddon grade 2 or axonotmesis injury, in which a transection of the axon occurs but the endoneurium remains intact. Wallerian degeneration occurs distal to the lesion, and a full and spontaneous recovery results within 2 to 3 months. Motor, sensory, and autonomic nerve dysfunction is complete at the time of injury.

A Sunderland third degree injury corresponds to an axonotmesis or clinical neurotmesis in which endoneurial damage occurs but fascicular patterns remain intact. Some lesions are reversible, whereas others are irreversible. The reversibility of the injury is dependent on the number of axons damaged and the extent of the fibrotic process within the funiculi.

A Sunderland fourth degree injury is a neuroma in continuity, resulting in fascicular disorganization with no gross retraction of the nerve ends with the epineurium intact. Spontaneous recovery cannot be expected, and this represents a clinical neurotmesis.

A Sunderland fifth degree injury corresponds to a Seddon grade 3 neurotmesis injury, in which there is a severance of the nerve with retraction of the ends and loss of anatomic continuity.

## PHYSICAL EXAMINATION

Clinical evaluation of a brachial plexus injury in an athlete must be performed in a careful and meticulous fashion. The localization and classification of lesions can be accomplished through a thorough and systematic physical examination. The trainer, physical therapist, and physician must be aware that athletes tend to underreport symptoms and/or injuries both at the preparticipation physical and during the on-field evaluation. To minimize loss of time from the sport, an aggressive approach to diagnosis and treatment is necessary.

The physical evaluation should begin with a brief but comprehensive musculoskeletal examination, including an evaluation of the head, neck, shoulders, elbows, wrists, and hands. The active and passive range of motion of the neck, shoulders, elbows, wrists, and fingers should be measured and recorded. The examination of the cervical spine is critical in differentiating between a cervical spine and a brachial plexus injury. The bony elements and paraspinal musculature should be evaluated for tenderness and the presence of paraspinal muscle spasm. Any pain evoked during palpation or range of motion of the cervical spine should be carefully noted. Provocative tests, such as the Spurling's maneuver, may be useful in the diagnosis of a cervical spine injury.

The shoulder should be evaluated to determine whether there is any evidence of acute or chronic instability that can contribute to brachial plexus pathology. The scapula should be observed at rest, as well as while the patient is pushing up against a wall. Any evidence of scapular winging should be noted that is due to either weakness of the serratus anterior or, occasionally, the trapezius. The clavicle should be palpated in its entirety to determine whether there is an acute fracture or whether exuberant callus formation has occurred.

A complete neurologic examination, including evaluation of motor strength, sensation, and deep tendon reflexes, must be performed. A thorough motor examination can often define the site of a lesion and differentiate between a root injury, preganglionic lesion, postganglionic lesion, diffuse plexus involvement, and peripheral nerve problem. Motor strength should be recorded using standard grading systems. Sensory examination should include an assessment of two-point discrimination, as well as light touch and pin-prick. The presence of Horner's syndrome (ptosis, miosis, anhidrosis, enophthalmos) should be noted by examination of the face, indicating a preganglionic lesion of T1.

A thorough vascular examination, including both venous and arterial functions, should be performed. The close proximity of the elements of the brachial plexus to the axillary vessels makes combined injuries possible, particularly with penetrating trauma.

## HIGH VELOCITY INJURIES

High velocity injuries are rare in sports, usually resulting instead from a motorcycle or motor vehicle accident or a fall from a height. These injuries are the result of severe traction on the plexus caused by forcible displacement of the head and shoulder away from one another. High velocity traction injuries are usually root avulsions, with the involved levels determined by the position of the upper extremity at the time of impact. Adduction results in injury to the upper roots. Abduction and extension results in injury to the entire plexus, and overhead abduction results in lower root injury.

Root avulsions are often accompanied by other significant injuries, including head injuries. Examination reveals motor and sensory deficits attributable to the involved roots. Cervical spine films may show transverse process fractures.[34] Myelography and magnetic resonance imaging may be used to show evidence of root avulsion, such as traumatic meningoceles.[43,55,65]

Histamine skin testing may be used as an adjunct test to differentiate between pre- and postganglionic lesions.[8,34,35] Histamine skin testing produces a normal three-phase response. The injection of 1% solution of histamine acid phosphate intradermally results in local vasal dilatation, whealing, and flare formation in the normal state. The vasodilatation and whealing are due to local effects of the histamine. The flare reaction is due to vasodilatation mediated through the sensory root ganglion and its distal afferent axons. Postganglionic injury disrupts the distal afferent axons, and the flare response is blocked. In preganglionic lesions the distal afferent axons are intact, and the flare response is present. A normal three-phase response indicates the presence of a preganglionic lesion, suggesting a poor prognosis.[34]

Sensory nerve conduction velocities and sensory nerve action potentials to the anesthetic regions are normal in these preganglionic lesions, as the dorsal root ganglion in distal afferent axons is intact. The EMG of the posterior cervical muscles, as well as serratus anterior and rhomboids, will reveal denervation patterns.

Recovery of function does not occur in root avulsions. Present surgical treatment consists primarily of muscle transfers with or without arthrodesis, although attempts at microsurgical repair may prove beneficial in the future. Associated postganglionic injury that may recover and reduce the extent of reconstruction required to obtain optimal function is a primary reason for delaying reconstruction. Early aggressive rehabilitation to maintain joint motion is important for obtaining optimal results.

## UPPER TRUNK BRACHIAL PLEXOPATHY

### BURNER OR STINGER SYNDROME

Burners, otherwise known as stingers, cervical nerve pinch injuries, and upper trunk brachial plexus injuries, are a unilateral upper extremity neurologic injury that frequently occur in contact sports, most notably football.[12,13,25,27,47] Clarke reported an incidence of 2.2 brachial plexus injuries per 100 players per year over a 4-year period.[14] Approximately 50% of collegiate-level football players sustain a burner during their career, and 30% of these players sustain their first injury in high school.[13] Warren noted a similar incidence among professional football players.[60]

The burner syndrome receives its name from the characteristic symptoms described by the affected athlete. Injury usually occurs while tackling, thus defensive and specialty team players are most commonly affected. Typically, following a blow to the head or neck, the athlete notices a sharp burning shoulder pain that often radiates to the ipsilateral arm and hand. The pain and paresthesias are not dermatomal in distribution and usually resolve within 1 to 2 minutes. The athlete will try to "shake off" the injury to restore feeling. Weakness may be present at the time of injury, with the athlete supporting the injured extremity while leaving the field. Weakness is usually transitory and resolves within minutes. Conversely, weakness may not develop for hours or several days after an injury, necessitating repeated postinjury neurologic examinations. Weakness, when present, involves the deltoid, biceps, supraspinatus, infraspinatus, and occasionally the supinator, brachioradialis, and pronator teres. Five percent to 10% of these injuries are more serious, causing a neurologic deficit that lasts several hours or longer.[4] A true burner is not generally associated with neck pain or significant restriction of neck mobility. The presence of neck pain should raise concern about the possibility of cervical spine fracture or more serious injury. Tenderness over the trapezius in the supraclavicular region may be found on examination lasting several days postinjury. Chrisman and colleagues reported a 9.5% decrease in lateral neck flexion, which may be related to trapezial tenderness and may go clinically undetected.[11]

There has been conflicting information regarding the pathogenetic mechanism and location of the injury along the course of the brachial plexus. This controversy concerns whether the lesion occurs in the brachial plexus* or at the root level.[1,11,45,50,63] The C5 and C6 levels are most commonly affected, indicating that the lesion will involve these root levels or the upper trunk of the brachial plexus. Three predominant mechanisms have been postulated. One mechanism involves a player making contact at the head and shoulder, with the head forced into lateral flexion while the shoulder is depressed away from the head and neck. The neurologic injury occurs on the side where shoulder depression occurs and has been attributed to a traction injury of the brachial plexus.† A second mechanism involves a direct blow to the supraclavicular region, causing direct compression of the brachial plexus.[1,2,6,36,50] A third mechanism has been attributed to cervical hyperextension and lateral flexion, causing ipsilateral foraminal compression of the nerve roots.[1,2,26,40]

Chrisman and colleagues investigated 22 players with a nerve pinch syndrome.[11] They noted that weakness persisted in some for more than 1 year. They concluded that the injury was a sprain of the cervical spine, with mild stretching of the nerve roots caused by a lateral flexion injury of the neck. They noted that a player of average build and flexibility was more prone to a lateral sprain than was an individual who was either short and thick-necked, or limber and long-necked.

Clancy and colleagues reported 13 cases of upper trunk brachial plexus injuries and classified them according to Seddon's criteria.[13] A grade I injury was an injury that resolved within 2 weeks. A grade II injury was classified as an injury that lasted greater than 2 weeks but resolved by 1 year. A grade III injury was defined as an injury in which the motor and sensory deficit persisted beyond 1 year with no clinical improvement. The

---

*References 4, 11, 13, 18, 36, 47, 50, 63.
†References 1, 2, 6, 12, 13, 25, 26.

mechanism of injury was a downward or backward blow to the ipsilateral shoulder with the neck flexed laterally away from the site of injury. EMG studies were performed on 10 players in an effort to pinpoint the location of the neural injury.[13,47] On the basis of a lack of involvement of the cervical paraspinal muscles, rhomboids, and serratus anterior muscles (which receive their innervation from proximal to Erb's point), the authors reported that the burner lesion was located in the upper trunk of the brachial plexus. They concluded that the mechanism of injury was traction on the brachial plexus.

Poindexter and Johnson performed electrodiagnostic studies on seven football players with the burner syndrome.[45] Six of the seven players had electrodiagnostic findings consistent with a C6 lesion. The researchers postulated that the mechanism of injury was an acute cervical flexion or extension injury.

Spear and Bassett reported on the "prolonged burner syndrome" in six players over the course of one football season.[50] Three of the six athletes had abnormal EMGs. Two of these three athletes had electrodiagnostic studies demonstrating evidence of C5 or C6 radiculopathy. The authors postulated that the traction injury was probably the most common cause of these injuries among football players, but they noted that some degree of direct compression may be associated with most of the injuries.

Markey and colleagues reported 32 cases of upper trunk brachial plexopathies in football players at the U.S. Military Academy.[36] Peripheral nerve injuries (axillary, musculocutaneous, suprascapular, thoracodorsal), as well as brachial plexus injuries, were noted. Electrophysiologic studies confirmed the location of the lesion to be at Erb's point in the upper trunk of the brachial plexus, with involvement of the accessory nerve at the superficial area in the neck. The authors hypothesized that compression of the fixed brachial plexus between the shoulder pad and the superior medial scapula, when the pad was pushed into the area of Erb's point at which the brachial plexus is most superficial, was a more common mechanism of injury.

Meyer and colleagues noted that players with an abnormal Torg ratio (less than 0.8) had a 3-times increased risk of incurring burners.[40] Linebackers and linemen were noted to have a higher incidence of burners. This was only applicable to the extension-compression mechanism and did not apply to the traction or direct compression mechanism. The level of cervical stenosis did not correlate with the position. Forty-five percent of players in this study who sustained burners had recurrent episodes of burners.

Clancy has classified brachial plexus injuries based on the duration of motor weakness and has paralleled Seddon's classification of nerve injuries.[12,25] Grade I injuries are the most common brachial plexus injuries, with a transitory loss of motor and sensory function that lasts from minutes to hours and completely resolves within 2 weeks. This represents a neurapraxia or physiologic interruption of nerve function. This may be due to edema or demyelinization of the axon without intrinsic axonal disruption, leading to a conduction block at the site of injury. The function returns as the edema resolves or when remyelinization is completed, usually within 2 or 3 weeks of injury. There is a complete return of strength. EMG studies at 2 to 3 weeks are normal.

Grade II injuries exhibit motor weakness lasting more than 2 weeks but with eventual full clinical recovery. Some athletes demonstrate weakness at the time of injury, whereas others may not exhibit weakness for several days. This is consistent with the work of Denny-Brown and Brenner.[15-17] There appears to be a two-phase recovery, with return of 80% to 90% of strength and endurance in 6 weeks and full recovery by 6 months. This pattern suggests a combined neurapraxia and axonotmesis. Wallerian degeneration of the distal axon is responsible for the delay in complete recovery, as axon regeneration requires as long as 6 months in this region. EMG changes at 3 weeks postinjury reveal evidence of muscle denervation with decreased motor unit potentials, fibrillations, and positive sharp waves. After complete clinical recovery, there may continue to be EMG changes (most commonly large motor unit potentials).

Grade III injuries are the rarest. Athletes who suffer these types of injuries continue to exhibit motor and sensory loss at 1 year postinjury, without clinical improvement. This represents a neurotmesis, with axonal regeneration frequently impossible because of the extent of injury. EMGs show evidence of denervation at 3 weeks postinjury, and again at 3 months, without evidence of recovery. Differentiation of axonotmesis from neurotmesis is important in determining the prognosis of the injury and the course of treatment. A grade III injury may benefit from operative intervention at or before 3 months.

Management of the athlete with a brachial plexus injury is based on clinical presentation. On-field evaluation includes motor and sensory examination. Weakness and anesthesia will persist while the pain is present but will usually resolve rapidly after the pain subsides. The supraspinatus, infraspinatus, deltoid, and biceps are the muscles most often involved. Elbow flexion and shoulder flexion usually return first, followed by shoulder external rotation and abduction. Sensory deficits are usually patchy and are most often present over the lateral shoulder. Persistent anesthesia is uncommon. Neck pain or loss of neck motion is uncommon in brachial plexus injuries and should raise concern about a possible cervical spine injury. Bilateral upper extremity burning dysesthesias may also represent a more significant cervical spine injury.[37]

If the athlete demonstrates no subjective pain or loss of neck motion, then testing of the shoulder rotators, deltoid, biceps, and triceps against resistance is performed. If the athlete's pain and subjective weakness have resolved and if no weakness is shown on examination, then return to play is allowed. The athlete must be examined again after the game and during the following week since weakness may be delayed. Routine cervical spine films, including anteroposterior, lateral (neutral, flexion, and extension), oblique, and open-mouth odontoid views, are recommended for athletes sustaining their first brachial plexus injury. Athletes with persistent pain or weakness beyond 2 weeks (grade II injury) should have routine cervical spine films and an EMG at 3 weeks postinjury to identify the site of the lesion. Evidence of a nerve root injury should prompt further study to rule out a disk herniation.

Treatment of grade I and II injuries involves removal of the athlete from participation as long as symptoms or weakness to manual muscle testing persist. The athlete is placed on a neck and shoulder strengthening program as soon as tolerated. Return to contact sports is based on return of strength and endurance of the shoulder muscles to normal, as compared with the contralateral, uninjured side. EMG studies in grade II injuries may show persistent changes even after return of strength and are not useful for determining return to play. Bergfeld and colleagues demonstrated that in players with brachial plexus injuries who initially had abnormal EMGs and neurologic deficits, 80% would still have abnormal EMGs at an average follow up of 4.25 years despite return to sports participation.[7,63] With return to football, use of a neck roll to prevent lateral flexion and posterior extension—and wearing built-up shoulder pads—may reduce the incidence of recurrent burners. Athletes with multiple burners may continue to participate as long as there is no loss of strength. Weakness should preclude participation until strength returns to normal. Stopping contact sports will eliminate further burners, but a return to play even after a prolonged period of nonparticipation is frequently associated with their recurrence.

Initial treatment of grade III injuries parallels treatment of the lesser injuries. Return to contact sports is prohibited because of the continued weakness.

## COMPRESSION INJURIES

Compression of the brachial plexus in association with athletic activities arises from both extrinsic and intrinsic factors.

Pack palsy or backpack paralysis represents an injury to the brachial plexus or its branches and is generally believed to be due to extrinsic compression of the plexus.[30,34,61] Ninety-four percent of the brachial plexus lesions in Hirasawa and Sakakida's series resulted from backpack paralysis.[30] The shoulder straps on a heavy pack create a compressive force on the plexus against the clavicle or first rib. The backward pull of a heavy pack on the shoulder girdle, which places traction on the plexus, has also been postulated as a contributing factor. Either mechanism is consistent with the studies of Denny-Brown that show that prolonged compression or low-grade traction can disrupt nerve function, which can be subsequently recovered.[15-17]

Pack palsy typically results in weakness involving a significant portion of the brachial plexus, or the injury may be restricted to the axillary or radial nerves. The clinical picture is one of profound weakness in the muscle groups involved. The condition is rarely painful, and sensory changes are not prominent.

Treatment of pack palsy is nonoperative, with an excellent prognosis. Hirasawa and Sakakida describe the complete clinical recovery of all 90 patients in their series, with "good results" following the use of range of motion and strengthening exercises within 3 months.[1]

Fractures of the clavicle with acute, displaced fragments; excessive callus formation[22,39,41]; or hypertrophic nonunions[32] may result in intrinsic brachial plexus compression.

Treatment of an acute clavicle fracture with a figure-eight bandage may result in brachial plexus compression. Repeat neurovascular evaluation of athletes with clavicle fractures is mandatory to avoid serious neurovascular compromise.[31-64] Adjustment or removal of the figure-eight strap is necessary if symptoms suggest potential compression of the brachial plexus. If symptoms are not relieved by removal of the figure-eight bandage, the possibility of fracture fragment encroachment on the brachial plexus and its associated vasculature should be evaluated and treated. This may require open reduction and internal fixation with decompression of the brachial plexus to allow safe and uncomplicated healing.

Exuberant callus formation may result in brachial plexus compression as clavicle fracture healing matures about the third week. The treatment involves resection of the excessive callus, followed by postoperative rehabilitation.

Hypertrophic nonunions producing brachial plexus symptoms generally involve the middle one third of the clavicle, compressing the plexus between the clavicle and the first and second ribs. The medial cord is usually involved, producing ulnar nerve symptoms.[39] Treatment consists of open reduction and internal fixation with bone grafting or partial excision of the clavicle.

Cervical ribs have also been implicated in brachial plexus compression.[46]

## ACUTE BRACHIAL NEUROPATHY

Acute brachial neuropathy is a clinical entity of unknown etiology that must be considered in the differential diagnosis of shoulder pain in the athlete. Acute brachial neuropathy[28,29] is described in the literature by the names serum brachial neuritis,[3,20,24,42] multiple neuritis,[10] localized neuritis of the shoulder girdle,[51] acute brachial radiculitis,[19,58] neuralgic amyotrophy,[21,44,59] shoulder girdle syndrome,[38,44] paralytic brachial neuritis,[5,23,33,35,62] Parsonage-Turner syndrome,[44] and brachial plexus neuropathy.[5,9,35,49] Burnard first described this syndrome among the servicemen in the second New Zealand expeditionary force.[10] Hershman and colleagues have described it in five athletes.[29]

The etiology of acute brachial neuropathy is unknown, and the syndrome often occurs sporadically. It has variously been related to trauma, exercise, surgery, infection, immunization, and genetics. Acute brachial neuropathy is characterized by constant, severe shoulder pain that is present at rest and responds poorly to analgesics. The onset of pain is sudden and may awaken a patient. Acute brachial neuropathy occurs acutely or subacutely in association with sports and is typically not related to a specific, traumatic event. The pain may last for several hours to weeks. Shoulder and elbow motion aggravate the pain. Shoulder adduction with elbow flexion is the most comfortable resting posture. Radiation of pain below the elbow suggests diffuse involvement of the brachial plexus or involvement of the lower plexus.

Weakness or paralysis usually appears within 2 weeks of pain onset. Weakness or paralysis may accompany the onset of pain but is more commonly noted as the pain is resolving; it may become apparent during athletic activity. Weakness or paralysis is characteristically patchy in distribution and involves lower motor neurons without a precise motor nerve, radicular, or nerve trunk pattern. The most commonly affected muscle is the deltoid, followed by the supraspinatus and infraspinatus, serratus anterior, biceps, triceps, and wrist and finger extensors.[29,56] Sensory deficits are minimal, usually limited to a small area over the lateral shoulder or radial surface of the forearm, and do not parallel the motor changes. Changes in deep tendon reflexes depend on the severity of muscle weakness, and decreased biceps and triceps reflexes are most common. Bilateral involvement is common and usually asymmetric, with subclinical involvement of one side requiring EMG evaluation for diagnosis.

EMG yields variable data, finding involvement of a single muscle to diffuse involvement of the brachial plexus. The EMG findings are primarily fibrillation potentials in affected muscles, and nerve conduction changes consist of decreases in amplitudes of motor and sensory nerve conduction in involved nerves. Nerve conduction velocities and motor distal latencies are not affected to any significant degree. The principal findings in the EMG studies of acute brachial neuropathy that differ from traumatic upper trunk injuries are involvement of muscles not innervated by the upper trunk (trapezius, serratus anterior, diaphragm); involvement of muscles innervated by a single or two peripheral nerves; involvement of a single muscle or sparing of other muscles innervated by the same portion of the trunk or plexus; severe motor involvement, with sparing of sensory functions in the same portion of the plexus; and unequal involvement of sensory nerves in the same portion of the plexus.[29] These findings have led some to consider acute brachial neuropathy to be a multiple axon loss—mononeuropathy multiplex—rather than a brachial plexopathy.

The treatment of acute brachial neuropathy is divided into two phases. Phase I is from onset to resolution of pain, with treatment consisting of rest, support with a sling, and analgesia. Activity may exacerbate the pain, but if tolerated, general range of motion exercises are performed to maintain joint motion. Phase II begins after the resolution of pain and consists of bilateral complete upper body strengthening, including scapular rotators. This total upper extremity approach is important because of the frequent subclinical involvement of muscles.

Return to normal function occurs in 75% of patients within 2 years and 90% of patients within 3 years.[57] Recovery usually begins within 1 to 2 months, with upper trunk lesions, unilateral lesions, or incomplete lesions progressing more rapidly than lower trunk lesions, bilateral lesions, or complete lesions. Mild residual deficits are relatively frequent, and scapular winging, when present initially, is likely to persist.[29]

Criteria for return to play can be guided by strength recovery. The patient may be allowed to return to play when strength equals that of the uninjured side or when strength has reached a plateau that is adequate for safe participation. Absolute strength parity may be unobtainable because of a persistent neurologic deficit. This requires that each case be considered individually. Recurrences are rare and are characterized by less severe symptoms of shorter duration.

## SUMMARY

Brachial plexus injuries, although rare in noncontact sports, are common in contact sports, especially American football. An understanding of the anatomy and neurophysiology is essential for establishing an accurate diagnosis and prognosis in brachial plexus injuries. Although severe and permanent disabilities may result, complete clinical recovery from sports-related brachial plexus injuries is generally the rule. During the recovery period, the cornerstone of treatment is protection from further injury—by avoiding contact sports and engaging in rehabilitation through range of motion and strengthening exercises. Safe return to athletic competition may be allowed when clinical recovery (normal sensation and strength parity) is achieved, despite mild changes in neurophysiologic studies.

## References

1. Albright J, Moses J, Feldick H et al: Non fatal cervical spine injuries in interscholastic football, *JAMA* 236:1243, 1976.
2. Albright JP, McAuley E, Martin RK et al: Head and neck injuries in college football: an eight-year analysis, *Am J Sports Med* 13:147-152, 1985.
3. Allen IM: The neurological complications of serum treatment: with report of a case, *Lancet* 2:1128-1131, 1931.
4. Archambault JL: Brachial plexus stretch injury, *Injury* 31:256-260, 1983.
5. Bale JF Jr, Thompson JA, Petajan JH et al: Childhood brachial plexus neuropathy, *J Pediatr* 95:741-742, 1979.
6. Bateman JE: Nerve injuries about the shoulder in sports, *J Bone Joint Surg* 49A:785-792, 1967.
7. Bergfeld JA, Hershman E, Wilbourn A: Brachial plexus injury in sports: a five-year follow up, *Orthop Trans* 12:743-744, 1988.
8. Bonney G: The value of axon responses in determining the site of a lesion in traction injuries of the brachial plexus, *Brain* 77:588-609, 1954.
9. Bufalini C, Pescatori G: Posterior cervical electromyography in the diagnosis and prognosis of brachial plexus injuries, *J Bone Joint Surg* 51B:627-631, 1969.
10. Burnard ED, Fox TG: Multiple neuritis of shoulder girdle: report of nine cases occurring in second New Zealand expeditionary force, *N Z Med J* 41:243-247, 1942.
11. Chrisman OD, Snook GA, Stanitis JM et al: Lateral-flexion neck injuries in athletic competition, *JAMA* 192:117-119, 1965.
12. Clancy WG: Brachial plexus and upper extremity peripheral nerve injuries. In Torg JS, editor: *Athletic injuries to the head, neck, and face*, Philadelphia, 1982, Lea & Febiger.
13. Clancy WG, Brand R, Bergfeld J: Upper trunk brachial plexus injuries in contact sports, *Am J Sports Med* 5:209, 1977.
14. Clarke K: An epidemiologic view. In Torg JS, editor: *Athletic injuries to the head, neck, and face*, ed 2, St Louis, 1991, Mosby–Year Book.
15. Denny-Brown D, Brenner C: Lesion in peripheral nerve resulting from compression by spring clip, *Arch Neurol Physiol* 52:1, 1944.
16. Denny-Brown D, Brenner C: Paralysis of nerve induced by direct pressure and by tourniquet, *Arch Neurol Physiol* 51:1, 1944.
17. Denny-Brown D, Doherty M: Effects of transient stretching of the peripheral nerve, *Arch Neurol Psychiatry* 54:116, 1945.
18. Di Benedetto M, Markey K: Electrodiagnostic localization of traumatic upper trunk brachial plexopathy, *Arch Phys Med Rehabil* 65:15, 1984.
19. Dixon GJ, Dick TBS: Acute brachial radiculitis: course and prognosis, *Lancet* 2:707-708, 1945.
20. Doyle JB: Neurologic complications of serum sickness, *Am J Med Sci* 185:484-492, 1933.
21. England JD, Sumner AJ: Neurologic amyotrophy: an increasingly diverse entity, *Muscle Nerve* 10:60-68, 1967.

22. Enker SH, Murphy KK: Brachial plexus compression by excessive callus formation secondary to a fractured clavicle: a case report, *Mt Sinai J Med* 37:678-682, 1972.
23. Evans HW: Paralytic brachial neuritis, *NY J Med* 65:2926-2928, 1965.
24. Flaggman PD, Kelly JJ Jr: Brachial plexus neuropathy: an electrophysiologic evaluation, *Arch Neurol* 37:160-164, 1980.
25. Freeman TR, Clancy WG Jr: Brachial plexus injuries. In Andrews JR, Wilk KE, editors: *The athlete's shoulder*, New York, 1994, Churchill Livingstone.
26. Funk FJ, Wells RE: Injuries of the cervical spine in football, *Clin Orthop* 109:50-58, 1975.
27. Griffin LY, editor: *Orthopaedic knowledge update: sports medicine*, Rosemont, Ill, 1994, American Academy of Orthopaedic Surgeons.
28. Hershman EB: Brachial plexus injuries, *Clin Sports Med* 9:311-329, 1990.
29. Hershman EB, Wilbourn AJ, Bergfeld J: Acute brachial neuropathy in athletes, *Am J Sports Med* 17:655-659, 1989.
30. Hirasawa Y, Sakakida K: Sports and peripheral nerve injuries, *Am J Sports Med* 11:420, 1983.
31. Howard FM, Shafer SJ: Injuries to the clavicle with neurovascular complications: a study of 14 cases, *J Bone Joint Surg* 47A:1335-1346, 1965.
32. Kay SP, Eckardt JJ: Brachial plexus palsy secondary to clavicular nonunion: a case report and literature survey, *Clin Orthop* 206:219-222, 1986.
33. Kennedy WR, Resch JA: Paralytic brachial neuritis, *Lancet* 86:459-462, 1966.
34. Leffert RD: Brachial plexus injuries, *N Engl J Med* 291:1059-1066, 1974.
35. Magee KR, DeJong RN: Paralytic brachial neuritis: discussion of clinical features with review of 23 cases, *JAMA* 174:1258-1262, 1960.
36. Markey KL, Di Benedetto MD, Curl WW: Upper trunk brachial plexopathy: the stinger syndrome, *Am J Sports Med* 21:650-655, 1993.
37. Maroon JC: "Burning hands" in football spinal cord injuries, *JAMA* 238:2049-2051, 1977.
38. Martin WA, Kraft GH: Shoulder girdle neuritis: a clinical and electrophysiological evaluation, *Mil Med* 139:21-25, 1974.
39. Matz SO, Welliver PS, Welliver DI: Brachial plexus neurapraxia complicating a comminuted clavicle fracture in a college football player, *Am J Sports Med* 17:581-583, 1989.
40. Meyer SA, Schulte KR, Callaghan JJ et al: Cervical spinal stenosis and stingers in collegiate football players, *Am J Sports Med* 22:158-166, 1994.
41. Miller DS, Boswick JA Jr: Lesions of the brachial plexus associated with fractures of the clavicle, *Clin Orthop* 64:144-149, 1969.
42. Miller HG, Stanton JB: Neurological sequelae of prophylactic inoculation, *Q J Med* 23:1-27, 1954.
43. Murphey F, Hartung W, Kirklin JW: Myelographic demonstration of avulsing injury of the brachial plexus, *Am J Roentgen* 58:102-105, 1947.
44. Parsonage MJ, Turner JWA: Neurologic amyotrophy: shoulder girdle syndrome, *Lancet* 1:973-978, 1948.
45. Poindexter D, Johnson E: Football, shoulder and neck injury: a study of the "stinger," *Arch Phys Med Rehabil* 65:601, 1984.
46. Rayan GM: Lower trunk brachial plexus compression neuropathy due to cervical rib in young athletes, *Am J Sports Med* 16:77-79, 1988.
47. Robertson W, Eichman P, Clancy W: Upper trunk brachial plexopathy in football players, *JAMA* 241:1480, 1979.
48. Seddon H: *Surgical disorders of the peripheral nerves*, Edinburgh, 1972, Churchill Livingstone.
49. Shaywitz BA: Brachial plexus neuropathy in childhood, *J Pediatr* 86:913-914, 1975.
50. Speer K, Bassett F: The prolonged burner syndrome, *Am J Sports Med* 18:591, 1990.

51. Spillane JD: Localized neuritis of shoulder girdle: report of 46 cases in MEF, *Lancet* 2:532-535, 1943.
52. Sunderland S: Mechanisms of cervical nerve root avulsion in injuries of the shoulder, *J Neurosurg* 41:705-714, 1974.
53. Sunderland S: *Nerve and nerve injuries,* ed 2, Edinburgh, 1978, Churchill Livingstone.
54. Takazawa H, Sudon, Aoki K et al: Statistical observation of nerve injuries in athletics, *Brain Nerve Injuries* 3:11, 1971 (in Japanese).
55. Tarlov IM, Day R: Myelography to help localized traction lesions of the brachial plexus, *Am J Surg* 88:266-271, 1954.
56. Taylor RA: Heredofamilial mononeuritis multiplex with brachial predilection, *Brain* 83:113-137, 1960.
57. Tsairis P, Dyck PJ, Mulder DW: Natural history of brachial plexus neuropathy: report on 99 patients, *Arch Neurol* 27:109-117, 1972.
58. Turner JWA: Acute brachial radiculitis, *BMJ* 2:592-594, 1944.
59. Turner JWA, Parsonage MJ: Neurologic amyotrophy (paralytic brachial neuritis): with special reference to prognosis, *Lancet* 2:209-212, 1957.
60. Warren R: Neurologic injuries in football. In Jordan BD, Tsairis P, Warren RS, editors: *Sports neurology,* Rockville, Md, 1989, Aspen Publishers.
61. White HH: Pack palsy: a neurological complication of scouting, *J Pediatr* 41:1001-1003, 1968.
62. Wiekers J, Mattson RH: Acute paralytic brachial neuritis: a clinical and electrodiagnostic study, *Neurology* 19:1153-1158, 1969.
63. Wilbourn AJ, Hershman EB, Bergfeld JA: Brachial plexopathies in athletes: the EMG findings, *Muscle Nerve* 9(suppl 5):254, 1986.
64. Yates DW: Complications of fractures of the clavicle, *Injury* 7:881-883, 1976.
65. Yeoman PN: Cervical myelography in traction injuries of the brachial plexus, *J Bone Joint Surg* 50B:253-260, 1968.

# Chapter 9

# Neck trauma

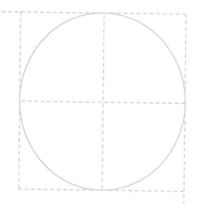

Alan G. Posta, Jr.
William G. Clancy, Jr.

A wide variety of cervical spine injuries may occur in the athlete. Athletic injuries to the cervical spine are not uncommon and represent a significant proportion of athletic injuries that produce permanent disability. During athletic competition the cervical spine may be injured in a variety of ways. Prompt recognition, appropriate assessment, transportation, and proper treatment are essential for the safe and timely return of the injured athlete to participation.

## EPIDEMIOLOGY

Cervical spine injuries may occur in any sport. Injuries resulting in spinal cord damage have been reported in football,* ice hockey,[80,108-110,112] gymnastics,[96,97,100,101] wrestling,[25,143] rugby,† trampolining,‡ and water sports.§ Football was the first sport to receive epidemiologic study because mortality data were available. Schneider[94] observed that "there is probably no experimental or research laboratory for human trauma better in the world than the football fields of our nation." Albright and colleagues[5] noted that 32% of freshmen college football players had abnormal cervical spine radiographs. Andrish and colleagues,[10] in a prospective study of football players at the U.S. Naval Academy during the 1974 season, reported a 15.6% incidence of neck injuries. Athletes who sustained one neck injury were 5 times more likely to sustain a recurrent injury compared with those with no history of cervical spine injuries. Schneider,[95] using injury data from 1959 to 1963, reported 56 cases (1.36

---

*References 18, 19, 30, 40, 57, 63, 68, 69, 94-97, 113, 119-131, 137.
†References 21, 64, 72, 86, 87, 90, 92, 93, 99, 100, 141, 142.
‡References 34, 36, 39, 47, 100, 106, 115, 116.
§References 1-3, 7, 26, 27, 31, 41, 42, 46, 55, 56, 65, 76, 81, 83, 88, 89, 91, 104, 111, 140.

cases per 100,000 participants) of cervical spine fracture, subluxation, or dislocation, and 30 cases (0.73 case per 100,000 participants) of permanent cervical quadriplegia. Torg and colleagues,[122] analyzing National Football Head and Neck Injury Registry (NFHNIR) data from 1971 to 1975, reported 259 cases (4.14 cases per 100,000 participants) of cervical spine fracture, subluxation, or dislocation, and 99 cases (1.58 cases per 100,000 participants) of permanent cervical quadriplegia. This represented a 204% increase in cervical spine fractures, subluxations, and dislocations, and a 116% increase in cases of cervical quadriplegia. In response to these data, spearing was outlawed in high school and college football in January 1976. Following these rule changes, Torg and colleagues[129] (using NFHNIR data from 1976 to 1987) reported a precipitous drop in the incidence of cervical spine fractures-subluxations-dislocations and permanent cervical quadriplegia on both the high school and college levels (Table 9). Albright and colleagues,[4] in a prospective study of head and neck injuries in college football, noted that 18% of players reported a neck injury over a 7-year study period, with 45% of these players experiencing at least transient neurologic symptoms or deficits. More recently, Cantu[19]—in a prospective study of permanent cervical cord injuries in football players from 1977 to 1989—reported an injury incidence of 0.62 case per 100,000 participants among junior high and high school players and 1.64 cases per 100,000 participants among college players.

Epidemiologic data have also recently been reported for ice hockey. Cervical spine injuries appear to represent a relatively new phe-

**Table 9**
**CERVICAL SPINE FRACTURE-SUBLUXATION-DISLOCATION***

|  | 1976 | 1987 |
|---|---|---|
| High School | 7.72 | 2.31 |
| College | 30.66 | 10.66 |

**PERMANENT CERVICAL QUADRIPLEGIA***

|  | 1976 | 1987 |
|---|---|---|
| High School | 2.24 | 0.73 |
| College | 10.66 | 0 |

* Rates are per 100,000 participants.

nomenon. Before 1984, there were no reported cervical spine injuries attributed to ice hockey in the English literature. In 1984, Tator[109] reported six cases of major spinal cord injury attributable to hockey that were treated in two major hospitals in Toronto between 1974 and 1981. By 1987, 117 hockey-related spinal injuries were reported. The actual incidence of permanent cervical quadriplegia in American high school ice hockey is 2.56 cases per 100,000 participants, compared with 0.62 to 0.73 case per 100,000 participants for American high school football.[18,19,24,129] The risk of permanent cervical quadriplegia may be 3 times greater in ice hockey than in football.[109,110] Of the cervical spine injuries studied by Tator, 83% occurred in the 11- to 30-year-old age group—with 52% of the players who suffered cervical spine injuries having spinal cord involvement.[109,110] Reynen and Clancy[80] have identified the introduction of the hockey helmet and face mask, the increased level of aggressive play, and "loose officiating," as three factors contributing to the increased incidence of cervical spine injuries in hockey. They advocate strict enforcement of the standing rules, as well as rule changes to increase the severity of penalty for dangerous play.

## MECHANISM OF INJURY

Historically, hyperflexion and hyperextension forces have been implicated as the primary mechanisms of injury in athletic cervical spine injuries. Schneider,[94,95] the first researcher to catalog head and neck injuries in football, concluded that hyperflexion resulted in the most severe cervical spine injuries. He also noted that hyperextension may cause cervical spine lesions that result in neurologic damage. Numerous reports have emphasized the role of these mechanisms in a variety of cervical spine injuries; cervical spine injuries with cord damage; and cervical spine fractures, subluxations, or dislocations.*

Recent literature, primarily the data from Torg and colleagues[113,119-131] and the NFHNIR, suggests that axial loading is the predominant mechanism of injury for athletic cervical spine injuries. Secondary forces—including hyperflexion, hyperextension, and rotation—may contribute to the injury pattern. Several authors—including Tator[109,111,112] (ice hockey, diving), Reynen and Clancy[80] (ice hockey), Scher[88] (diving), Torg[115,116] (trampolining), and Watkins[137] (football)—identify axial loading as the primary force responsible for athletic cervical spine injuries.

---

*References 7, 30, 40, 42, 52, 54-57, 60, 63-65, 72, 75, 77, 83, 87, 99, 104, 140, 141, 143.

Biomechanical research supports the notion of axial loading as the principal mechanism responsible for athletic cervical spine injuries. Mertz and colleagues,[66] Hodgson and Thomas,[51] and Sances and colleagues[85] applied axial loads to helmeted cadaver head-spine-trunk specimens and produced fractures of the lower cervical spine. Gosch and colleagues[43] examined three different injury mechanisms and concluded that axial compression produced cervical spine fractures and dislocations. White and Panjabi,[139] Maiman and colleagues,[61] and Roaf[82] demonstrated vertebral body fractures in the lower cervical spine caused by axial loading of isolated spinal units. Roaf investigated compression, flexion, extension, lateral flexion, rotation, and horizontal shear and was unable to produce a pure hyperflexion injury. Carter and Frankel[20] examined the hyperextension (guillotine) mechanism and concluded that this mechanism was invalid. Virgin,[135] using cineradiography, studied 16 helmeted football players and was unable to demonstrate any contact between the posterior rim of the helmet and the cervical vertebral spinous process. Bauze and Ardran[14] produced unilateral and bilateral facet dislocations without bony injury by applying axial loads to cadaveric spines.

Critical limits of compressive loads for the cervical vertebral bodies have been estimated to be approximately 3340 to 4450 N.[74,139] Several investigators have demonstrated that the greatest axial forces are applied to the cervical spine in slight flexion.[6,51,61] Torg and colleagues,[129] using the law of conservation of linear momentum, calculated the forces generated during a football head-on collision to be approximately 4000 to 8000 N. Bishop and Wells[14] reported that impact velocities in ice hockey as low as 1.8 m/sec produced compressive loads from C3 to C5 to 75% of failure in axial compression. The average speed of a sliding skater is 6.7 m/sec, whereas normal skating speed is approximately 9.4 to 12.2 m/sec.[102] Clearly, axial compressive forces exceeding critical load limits for failure may be generated during athletic competition.

The cervical spine in the neutral position is slightly extended because of the normal lordotic curve. Forces applied to the cervical spine are effectively dispersed by the intervertebral disks and paraspinal musculature. This energy absorption process is achieved through controlled spinal motion (Fig. 9-1). With 30 degrees of flexion, the cervical spine becomes a straight segmented column. When axial loads are applied, controlled spinal motion cannot be achieved. Resultant axially directed forces are transmitted directly to the intervertebral disks, ligamentous tissues, and bony elements. Continued energy input beyond maximum deformation limits causes failure of the intervertebral disks, ligaments, and bony elements—resulting in fractures, subluxations, dislocations, or fracture-dislocations (Fig. 9-2).

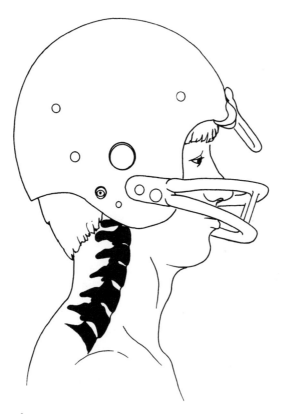

**Fig. 9-1.** When the neck is in a normal, upright, anatomic position, the cervical spine is slightly extended because of the natural cervical lordosis. (With permission from Torg JS et al: The epidemiologic, pathologic, biomechanical, and cinematographic analysis of football-induced cervical spine trauma, *Am J Sports Med* 18:50-57, 1990.)

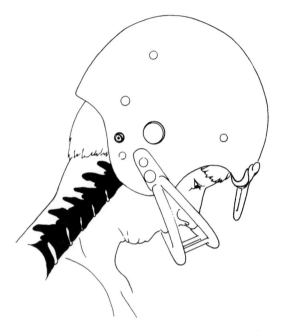

**Fig. 9-2.** When the neck is flexed slightly, to approximately 30 degrees, the cervical spine is straightened and converted into a segmented column. (With permission from Torg JS et al: The epidemiologic, pathologic, biomechanical, and cinematographic analysis of football-induced cervical spine trauma, *Am J Sports Med* 18:50-57, 1990.)

## CLASSIFICATION

Athletic cervical spine injuries encompass a broad spectrum and include the following injury patterns: (1) cervical strains and sprains; (2) brachial plexus injuries (see Chapter 8); (3) transient quadriplegia-cervical stenosis; (4) spinal cord injury; (5) spear tackler's spine; and (6) acute cervical spine fractures, subluxations, and dislocations.

### STRAINS AND SPRAINS

Cervical spine strains and sprains represent the most common athletic cervical spine injuries. Strains are defined as injuries to the muscle-tendon unit, whereas sprains represent ligamentous or capsular injuries. The cervical muscles most commonly involved are the sternocleidomastoid, trapezius, rhomboids, erector spinae, scalenes, and levator scapulae. Clinically the athlete may complain of pain that may be exacerbated by neck motion. Swelling, tenderness, and paraspinal muscle spasm may become apparent. Neurologic deficits are not present. The degree of injury may range from mild to severe. Cervical spine instability may result if significant ligamentous or capsular disruption occurs.

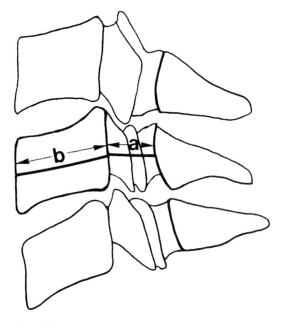

**Fig. 9-3.** The ratio of the spinal canal to the vertebral body is the distance from the midpoint of the posterior aspect of the vertebral body to the nearest point on the corresponding spinolaminar line (*a*) divided by the anteroposterior width of the vertebral body (*b*).

## TRANSIENT QUADRIPLEGIA-CERVICAL STENOSIS

Neurapraxia of the cervical spinal cord with transient quadriplegia is a clinical entity characterized by sensory changes that may be associated with motor paresis.[113,119,120] Sensory changes include burning pain, numbness, tingling, and loss of sensation. Motor changes may consist of weakness or complete paralysis involving both arms, both legs, or all four extremities. The episodes are transient and recovery usually occurs within 10 to 15 minutes but may take up to 36 to 48 hours. Neck pain is not present at the time of injury. Complete return of motor function and full, pain-free cervical spine motion is the rule. Routine radiographs of the cervical spine demonstrate no evidence of fracture, subluxation, or dislocation.

Torg and colleagues[113,119,120] have identified the association between cervical spinal stenosis and transient quadriplegia. Cervical stenosis is defined as one or more vertebrae having a canal/body ratio less than or equal to 0.8 (Fig. 9-3). Recent reports have documented the low predictive value of the Torg ratio, with 29% to 49% of asymptomatic college and professional football players having abnormal ratios.[49,67,73] However, 92% of all reported episodes of transient quadriplegia had abnormal Torg ratios.[118] Only 2 of 296 athletes who suffered cervical spine injuries associated with permanent neurologic sequelae had documented evidence of a previous episode of transient quadriplegia.[124] Athletes who experience an incidence of transient quadriplegia do not appear to be at increased risk for future clinical episodes or for the development of a permanent neurologic injury.

## SPINAL CORD INJURY

Spinal cord injuries in athletics are rare. Spinal cord injuries are either complete or incomplete. The severity of a spinal cord injury cannot be determined until spinal shock resolves (which is marked by the return of the bulbocavernosus reflex, usually within 48 hours). The Frankel classification is the most commonly used grading scale for evaluating patients with spinal cord injuries. (See the box below.) Prompt treatment of spinal cord injuries with methylprednisolone, initiated with a 30 mg/kg bolus followed by 5.4 mg/kg/hr infused over the next 23 hours, may result in significant motor and sensory improvement if administered within 8 hours of injury.[16]

### Complete

Complete spinal cord lesions are defined as complete loss of spinal cord function below the injury level. This is determined once spinal shock has resolved. The prognosis for a patient with a complete spinal cord injury is poor. Nerve root recovery at one or two levels below the injury level may occur.

### Incomplete

Incomplete spinal cord lesions can be divided into four types: (1) central cord syndrome, (2) Brown-Séquard syndrome, (3) anterior cord syndrome, and (4) posterior cord syndrome.

The central cord syndrome is the most common incomplete cord lesion. The central portion of the spinal cord is damaged, usually secondary to a hyperextension injury to the cervical spine in the setting of

---

**FRANKEL CLASSIFICATION OF SPINAL CORD INJURY PARALYSIS**

| | |
|---|---|
| Grade A | Complete; no motor or sensory function |
| Grade B | Incomplete; sensation intact only |
| Grade C | Incomplete; sensation intact with useless motor function |
| Grade D | Incomplete; sensation intact with useful motor function |
| Grade E | Normal; normal motor and sensory function |

cervical spondylosis. This syndrome is characterized by greater upper extremity (versus lower extremity) motor weakness. There may be associated sensory changes and bowel or bladder dysfunction. The patient with central cord syndrome has a fair prognosis. Bowel and bladder function generally returns. Neurologic recovery is usually greater in the lower extremities than in the upper extremities.

The Brown-Séquard syndrome is characterized by loss of ipsilateral motor function and by contralateral pain and temperature sensation. This syndrome is rare in athletes and may occur secondary to penetrating trauma. The patient with Brown-Séquard syndrome has a favorable prognosis for return of bowel, bladder, and ambulatory function.

The anterior cord syndrome represents an injury to the anterior two thirds of the spinal cord secondary to an ischemic injury in the distribution of the anterior spinal artery. This results in bilateral loss of motor function that is greater in the lower extremity than in the upper extremity. A patient with this syndrome has a generally poor prognosis.

The posterior cord syndrome is characterized by injury to the dorsal columns and usually results from an ischemic injury in the distribution of the spinal cord that is supplied by the posterior spinal artery. This results in loss of the senses of touch, vibration, and position. This syndrome occurs very rarely in athletes and may manifest itself clinically as a slap-foot gait.

## SPEAR TACKLER'S SPINE

Spear tackler's spine is a clinical entity marked by the following characteristics: (1) developmental narrowing of the cervical canal (Torg ratio less than 0.8); (2) persistent straightening or reversal of the normal cervical lordotic curve on erect, neutral, lateral radiographs; (3) concomitant preexisting posttraumatic radiographic abnormalities of the cervical spine; and (4) documented use of spear tackling techniques.[124] Twenty-seven percent of players identified with spear tackler's spine sustained permanent neurologic injuries.[124] Spear tackler's spine represents an absolute contraindication to participation in collision sports.

## CERVICAL SPINE FRACTURES-SUBLUXATIONS-DISLOCATIONS

Traumatic cervical spine injuries resulting in fractures, subluxations, and dislocations may represent stable or unstable injuries and may or may not be accompanied by neurologic compromise. Treatment is aimed at preventing neurologic injury, maintaining cervical spine alignment, achieving spinal stability, and beginning early rehabilitation. The cervical spine can be divided into three segments—upper (occiput to C2), middle (C3 to C4), and lower (C5 to C7) based on injury patterns.

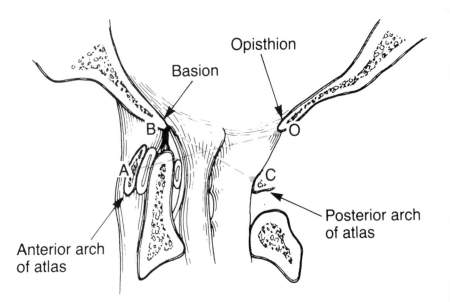

**Fig. 9-4.** Powers' ratio. If *BC:OA* is greater than 1, then an anterior atlantooccipital dislocation exists. Ratios less than 1 are normal except in posterior dislocations, associated fractures of the odontoid process or ring of the atlas, and congenital anomalies of the foramen magnum. (With permission from Jarrett PJ, Whitesides TE Jr: Injuries of the cervicocranium. In Browner BD, Jupiter JB, Levine AM, Trafton PG, editors: *Skeletal trauma,* vol 1, Philadelphia, 1992, WB Saunders.)

#### Upper cervical spine injuries

Atlantooccipital dislocations are rare in athletics and are usually fatal. The radiographic diagnosis is made on the neutral, lateral radiograph, with a Powers' ratio greater than 1 indicating an anterior atlantooccipital dislocation and less than 1 indicating a posterior atlantooccipital dislocation (Fig. 9-4).[78] Treatment consists of immediate halo application, followed by posterior spinal fusion from the occiput to the upper cervical spine (C1 or C2).

Occipital condyle fractures usually represent stable injuries. Treatment consists of simple orthotic immobilization. Rare cases of atlantooccipital instability may require occiput to C1 arthrodesis.

Fractures of the atlas have been classified into five major types: (1) anterior arch fractures, (2) posterior arch fractures, (3) lateral mass fractures, (4) Jefferson's (burst) fractures, and (5) transverse process fractures (Fig. 9-5).[53] Atlas fractures are decompressive lesions and are rarely associated with neurologic deficits unless they are accompanied by odontoid fractures or transverse ligament (atlantoaxial instability) ruptures. Anterior arch fractures, lateral mass fractures, and transverse

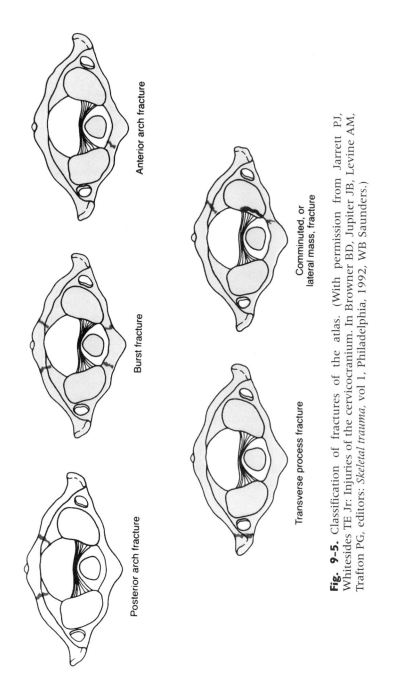

**Fig. 9-5.** Classification of fractures of the atlas. (With permission from Jarrett PJ, Whitesides TE Jr: Injuries of the cervicocranium. In Browner BD, Jupiter JB, Levine AM, Trafton PG, editors: *Skeletal trauma*, vol 1, Philadelphia, 1992, WB Saunders.)

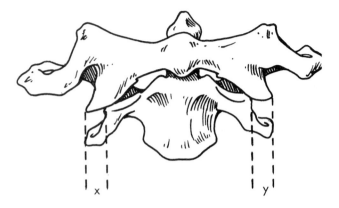

**Fig. 9-6.** Atlantoaxial offset. If $x + y$ is greater than 6.9 mm, transverse atlantal ligament rupture is implied.

process fractures usually represent stable injuries and may be managed by a halo or cervical orthosis until union is achieved. Isolated posterior arch fractures are stable injuries and may be managed with a cervical orthosis. Fifty percent of patients with posterior arch fractures have associated cervical spine injuries, including odontoid fractures and traumatic spondylolisthesis of the axis.[35,44,59,98] Treatment of Jefferson's (burst) fractures is based on the competency of the transverse ligaments. Atlantoaxial offset of greater than 6.9 mm, measured on the open-mouth radiograph, indicates transverse ligament rupture (Fig. 9-6).[103] Jefferson's fractures with atlantoaxial offset less than 6.9 mm are stable injuries and may be managed by a halo or cervical orthosis. There is no consensus on management of Jefferson's fractures with concomitant transverse ligament ruptures. Treatment consists of traction to achieve appropriate alignment, followed by halo vest immobilization. Posterior C1 to C2 arthrodesis may be indicated for residual atlantoaxial instability.

The stability of the atlantoaxial articulation is maintained by a ligamentous complex that consists primarily of the transverse ligament, with paired alar ligaments acting as secondary stabilizers. The apical, cruciate, and accessory ligaments and capsular ligaments of the facet joints provide stability to a much lesser degree (Figs. 9-7 and 9-8). Atlantoaxial instability is characterized by rupture of the transverse and alar ligaments and usually results from forced flexion of the neck. The radiographic diagnosis is made by examining the atlantodens interval (ADI) on lateral flexion-extension views (Fig. 9-9). The ADI is normally less than 3 mm in adults and 4 mm in children.[105] An ADI greater than 5 mm indicates ruptured and deficient transverse and accessory ligaments.[37,45,50,105,136] Treatment consists of posterior C1 to C2 arthrodesis.

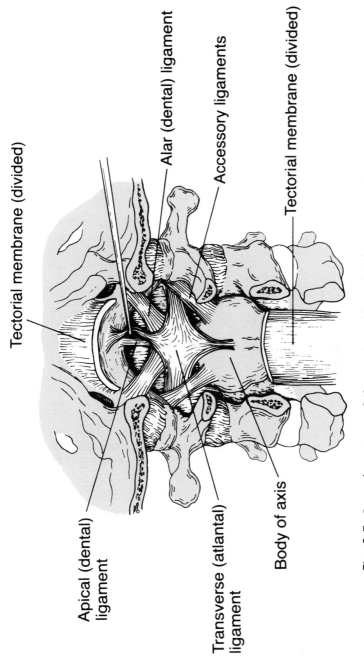

Tectorial membrane (divided)

Alar (dental) ligament

Accessory ligaments

Tectorial membrane (divided)

Apical (dental) ligament

Transverse (atlantal) ligament

Body of axis

**Fig. 9-7.** Coronal anatomy of the cervicocranium. (With permission from Jarrett PJ, Whitesides TE Jr: Injuries of the cervicocranium. In Browner BD, Jupiter JB, Levine AM, Trafton PG, editors: *Skeletal trauma*, vol 1, Philadelphia, 1992, WB Saunders.)

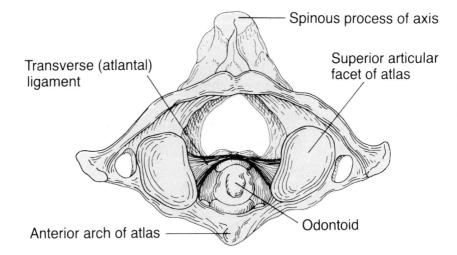

Spinous process of axis

Superior articular facet of atlas

Transverse (atlantal) ligament

Odontoid

Anterior arch of atlas

**Fig. 9-8.** The atlantoaxial articulation. (With permission from Jarrett PJ, Whitesides TE Jr: Injuries of the cervicocranium. In Browner BD, Jupiter JB, Levine AM, Trafton PG, editors: *Skeletal trauma*, vol 1, Philadelphia, 1992, WB Saunders.)

ADI

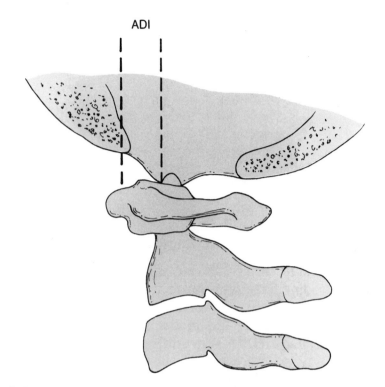

**Fig. 9-9.** Atlantodens interval (*ADI*). If the ADI is greater than 3 mm on flexion and extension roentgenograms, rupture of the transverse ligament is implied. If the ADI is greater than 5 mm, the accessory ligaments are also functionally incompetent. (With permission from Jarrett PJ, Whitesides TE Jr: Injuries of the cervicocranium. In Browner BD, Jupiter JB, Levine AM, Trafton PG, editors: *Skeletal trauma,* vol 1, Philadelphia, 1992, WB Saunders.)

C1 to C2 rotatory subluxation has been classified by Fielding into four types (Fig. 9-10).[38] This condition may occur in children secondary to an upper respiratory viral illness or, rarely, in athletes as a result of trauma. Patients may have complaints of neck pain, painful torticollis, and decreased range of motion of the cervical spine. The "wink sign" may be visible on the open-mouth radiograph. Subluxations in children usually are self-limited and resolve with a brief period of traction, followed by cervical collar immobilization. Acute deformities in adults are managed with skeletal traction, followed by halo vest immobilization. Surgical reduction and posterior C1 to C2 arthrodesis are reserved for cases of failed closed reduction, recurrent deformities, injuries associated with atlantoaxial instability, and injuries associated with neurologic deficit.

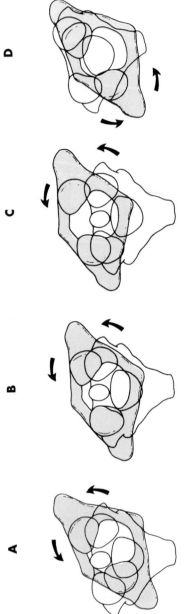

**Fig. 9-10.** Drawings showing the four types of rotatory subluxation. **A,** Type I: rotatory fixation with no anterior displacement and the odontoid acting as the pivot. **B,** Type II: rotatory fixation with anterior displacement of 3 to 5 mm and one lateral articular process acting as the pivot. **C,** Type III: rotatory fixation with anterior displacement of more than 5 mm. **D,** Type IV: rotatory fixation with posterior displacement. (With permission from Jarrett PJ, Whitesides TE Jr: Injuries of the cervicocranium. In Browner BD, Jupiter JB, Levine AM, Trafton PG, editors: *Skeletal trauma*, vol 1, Philadelphia, 1992, WB Saunders.)

Anderson and D'Alonzo have classified odontoid fractures into three types (Fig. 9-11).[9] The type I fracture is an avulsion of the alar ligaments off the tip of the odontoid and is a stable injury. Symptomatic treatment with a cervical orthosis is appropriate. The type II fracture is a fracture through the base of the odontoid process and is the most common type of odontoid fracture. Reported nonunion rates range from 15% to 85%.[44] Risk factors for nonunion include: (1) a displacement greater than 5 mm, (2) age over 40, (3) angulation greater than 10 degrees, and (4) improper treatment.[12,23] There is no consensus on management, which consists of reduction with traction followed by halo vest immobilization or primary posterior C1 to C2 arthrodesis for failed reductions and high-risk patients. Type III fractures extend into the body of C2 and are stable injuries. These can be managed with halo vest immobilization or a rigid cervical orthosis for nondisplaced fractures.

Traumatic spondylolisthesis of the axis (hangman's fracture) has been classified by Levine and Edwards into four types (Fig. 9-12).[58] Type I fractures demonstrate no angulation and less than 3 mm of displacement. This fracture is stable and may be managed with a cervical orthosis. Type II fractures demonstrate both angulation and displacement and are unstable injuries. Treatment consists of reduction with traction, followed by halo vest immobilization. Type IIA fractures have significant angulation with minimal translation. These also represent unstable injuries, and reduction is achieved by applying mild compression with extension, followed by halo vest immobilization. Type III fractures occur with concomitant unilateral or bilateral facet dislocations. Treatment consists of attempted closed reduction of the facet dislocation with halo traction. A successful reduction that can be maintained may be converted to halo vest immobilization. Failed closed reductions of the facet dislocation require open reduction with posterior C1 to C2 stabilization.

### Middle cervical spine injuries

Athletic injuries to the middle cervical spine (C3 to C4) are rare. Only 2.4% of the cervical spine fractures, subluxations, and dislocations documented by the NFHNIR occurred at the middle cervical spine.[126] Torg and colleagues[126] have described five types of injury patterns: (1) acute disk herniation, (2) anterior subluxation of C3 on C4, (3) unilateral facet dislocation, (4) bilateral facet dislocation, and (5) C4 body fracture. The response to axial loads in the middle cervical spine (C3 to C4) differs from that of the upper (C1 to C2) and lower (C5 to C7) segments. Injuries to the middle cervical spine involve predominantly the intervertebral disk, ligaments, and capsular structures (84%) and generally do not involve fracture of the bony elements (16%). Acute intervertebral disk herniations may be associated with episodes of transient quadriplegia. Reduction of anterior subluxation of C3 on C4 may be difficult to maintain. Reduction

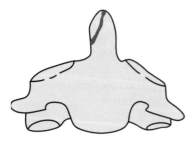

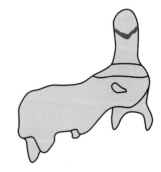

Type I

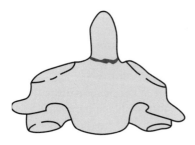

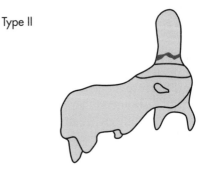

Type II

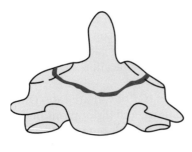

Type III

**Fig. 9-11.** Three types of odontoid fractures as seen in the anteroposterior and lateral planes. Type I is an oblique fracture through the upper part of the odontoid process itself. Type II is a fracture at the junction of the odontoid process with the vertebral body of the second cervical vertebra. Type III is really a fracture through the body of the atlas. (With permission from Anderson LD, D'Alonzo RT: Fractures of the odontoid process of the axis, *J Bone Joint Surg* 56A:1663-1674, 1974.)

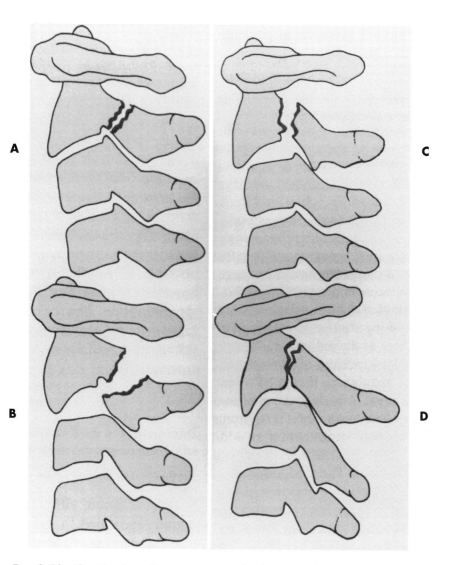

**Fig. 9-12.** Classification of traumatic spondylolisthesis of the axis. **A,** Type I injuries have a fracture through the neural arch with no angulation and as much as 3 mm of displacement. **B,** Type II fractures have both significant angulation and displacement. **C,** Type IIA fractures have shown minimum displacement, but there is severe angulation. **D,** Type III axial fractures combine bilateral facet dislocation between C2 and C3 with a fracture of the neural arch of the axis. (With permission from Levine AM, Edwards CC: Treatment of injuries in the C1-C2 complex, *Orthop Clin North Am* 17:31-44, 1986.)

of unilateral facet dislocation is difficult to obtain by skeletal traction and is best managed by closed reduction under general anesthesia. Reduction of bilateral facet dislocations is difficult to obtain by closed means and is best managed by open methods. Early, aggressive treatment yields the most favorable outcome for neurologic recovery.

**Lower cervical spine injuries**

Injuries to the lower cervical spine account for most of the fractures, subluxations, and dislocations sustained in athletic events. The decreasing ratio of canal diameter to cord diameter increases the likelihood that neural element compression will accompany cervical spine injuries. Patients must be evaluated for evidence of spinal deformity, instability, and neural element compression. Segmental instability, avulsion fractures, compression fractures, facet dislocations, burst fractures, and axial load teardrop fractures are described.

**Instability.** White and Panjabi[138,139] have determined a spine to be clinically unstable when one of three observations can be made: (1) there is potential for progressive encroachment or injury to neural structures, (2) there is potential for progressive displacement of the injured segment during the healing process, or (3) the injured segment of the spine will further angulate or displace under normal physiologic loading after complete healing has occurred. Radiographic instability, in an intact cervical spine without a vertebral body fracture, is defined as greater than 3.5 mm of horizontal translation or 11 degrees of angulation between adjacent vertebra (Fig. 9-13).[138,139] Treatment of unstable injuries of the lower cervical spine requires surgical stabilization.

**Avulsion injuries.** The clay shoveler's fracture represents an avulsion of the spinous process (most commonly of C7) and has been reported in power lifting and football.[48,71] This is a stable injury and may be treated with a cervical orthosis.

The extension teardrop fracture is an avulsion of the anterior-inferior corner of the vertebral body by the anterior longitudinal ligament. This lesion occurs most commonly at C2 but has been reported in the lower cervical spine.[97,121] This also represents a stable injury and may be treated with a cervical orthosis.

**Compression fractures.** Compression fractures by definition result in failure of the anterior column with an intact middle column, resulting in variable loss of anterior vertebral body height. Clinical management is based on the amount of compression and the presence of segmental instability. In general, isolated fractures with a loss of less than 25% of vertebral body height are stable and can be treated with a cervical orthosis. Compression fractures with a greater than 50% loss of vertebral body height often have concomitant segmental instability and require surgical stabilization.

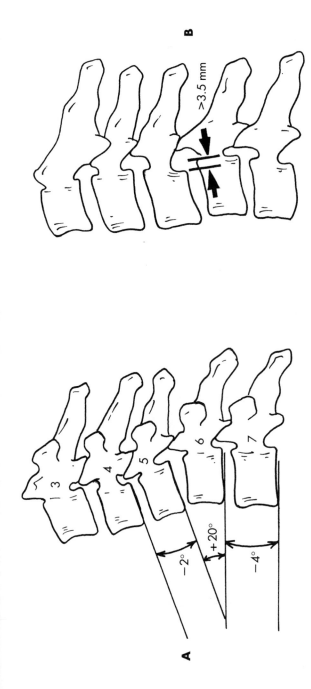

**Fig. 9-13.** White and colleagues have demonstrated that angular displacements of 11 degrees greater than those at the adjacent vertebral segments suggest instability secondary to posterior ligamentous disruption (**A**). In addition, vertebral body translation greater than 3.5 mm similarly suggests ligamentous instability, even in the absence of fracture (**B**).

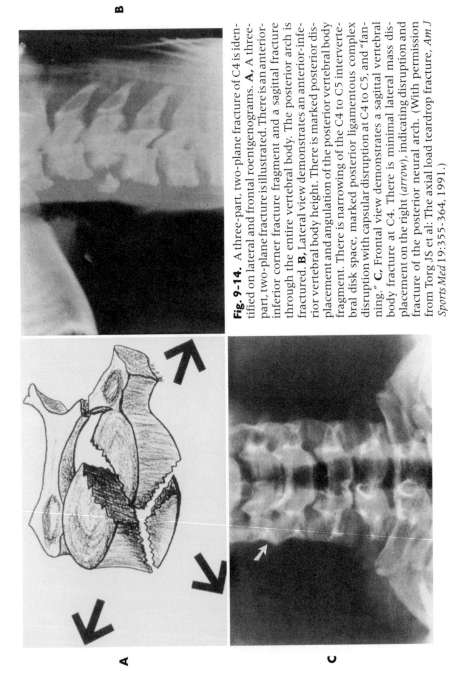

**Fig. 9-14.** A three-part, two-plane fracture of C4 is identified on lateral and frontal roentgenograms. **A,** A three-part, two-plane fracture is illustrated. There is an anterior-inferior corner fracture fragment and a sagittal fracture through the entire vertebral body. The posterior arch is fractured. **B,** Lateral view demonstrates an anterior-inferior vertebral body height. There is marked posterior displacement and angulation of the posterior vertebral body fragment. There is narrowing of the C4 to C5 intervertebral disk space, marked posterior ligamentous complex disruption with capsular disruption at C4 to C5, and "fanning." **C,** Frontal view demonstrates a sagittal vertebral body fracture at C4. There is minimal lateral mass displacement on the right (*arrow*), indicating disruption and fracture of the posterior neural arch. (With permission from Torg JS et al: The axial load teardrop fracture, *Am J Sports Med* 19:355-364, 1991.)

**Facet dislocations.** The radiographic diagnosis of a unilateral or bilateral facet dislocation may be observed on a lateral radiograph. Unilateral facet dislocations demonstrate approximately 25%—and bilateral facet dislocations demonstrate greater than 50%—displacement of the superior vertebrae on the inferior vertebrae. The "bow tie" sign may be viewed on the lateral radiograph. There is no consensus on the management of facet dislocations. The association between facet dislocations (most commonly bilateral facet dislocations) and concomitant disk herniation has been reported.* Reduction maneuvers may result in disk extrusion and potential neurologic compromise. Treatment consists of skeletal traction, followed by open reduction if unsuccessful. Successful closed reduction may be followed by halo vest immobilization or posterior arthrodesis. Magnetic resonance imaging (MRI) should be obtained to rule out a disk herniation in cases of neurologic deficit and difficult closed reductions. Anterior diskectomy and interbody fusion may be necessary if significant disk extrusion is present.

**Burst fractures.** Burst fractures involve injury to the anterior and middle columns and often the posterior elements and ligamentous structures. These lesions may have associated, severe spinal cord injuries. The immediate goal of management is to establish spinal alignment through skeletal traction. Patients with residual canal compromise and incomplete spinal cord injuries may undergo surgical decompression. Burst fractures are unstable injuries and usually require operative fixation.

**Axial load teardrop fractures.** Torg and colleagues[121] have described two fracture patterns associated with the axial load anteroinferior (teardrop) fracture: (1) the isolated fracture and (2) the three-part, two-plane fracture with an associated sagittal vertebral body fracture combined with a fracture of the posterior neural arch (Fig. 9-14). In the study by Torg and colleagues, 17% of patients with the isolated teardrop fracture had permanent neurologic deficits; 87% of patients with the three-part, two-plane fracture were rendered quadriplegic.[121]

## ON-FIELD EVALUATION AND MANAGEMENT OF CERVICAL SPINE INJURIES

On-field management of cervical spine injuries begins before the athletic event.[114,133,134] Prior planning can prevent catastrophic sequelae. The team physician or trainer should be identified as the person responsible

---

* References 8, 11, 15, 17, 28, 29, 32, 33, 70, 79, 84.

for on-field management of athletic cervical spine injuries, and this should be communicated to the players, coaches, and ancillary medical personnel. Arrangements should be made to ensure the presence of an ambulance and equipment necessary to initiate and maintain cardiopulmonary resuscitation (CPR). Athletes with cervical spine injuries should be transported to a medical facility with the equipment and staff—including appropriate orthopedic and neurosurgical personnel, as well as diagnostic radiographic modalities—to handle an emergency cervical spine injury. Several key pieces of emergency equipment must be available. These include a spine board, stretcher, rigid collar, and sand bags to immobilize the athlete. In football, bolt cutters or a sharp knife are necessary to facilitate face mask removal. A telephone must be available to aid in communication with the hospital emergency room—to alert them to the athlete's condition and estimated time of arrival so that adequate preparations can be made and to ensure continuity of care.

Prevention of further injury is the most important objective when managing athletic cervical spine injuries. It is estimated that 49% of patients sustain neurologic injuries after their initial injury has occurred.[62,132] Clinical evaluation of an athlete with a cervical spine injury must be performed in a careful and meticulous fashion. The initial assessment should include an accurate history. Documentation of the presence of neck pain, neurologic symptoms, loss of consciousness, preexisting cervical spine congenital anomalies, previous cervical spine trauma, and mechanism of injury is important.

In an ambulatory, conscious athlete the physical evaluation should begin with a brief but comprehensive musculoskeletal examination, including an evaluation of the head, neck, shoulders, elbows, wrists, and hands. The active and passive range of motion of the neck, shoulders, elbows, wrists, and fingers should be measured and recorded. The bony elements and paraspinal musculature should be evaluated for tenderness and the presence of paraspinal muscle spasm. Any pain evoked during palpation or range of motion of the cervical spine should be carefully noted. Provocative tests, such as the Spurling's maneuver, may be useful in the diagnosis of a cervical spine injury. A complete neurologic examination including evaluation of motor strength, sensation, and deep tendon reflexes must be performed. Cervical spine injury should be suspected in any athlete who complains of neck pain, numbness, weakness, or paralysis.

Management of unconscious athletes or those with suspected cervical spine injuries should begin with immobilization of the head and neck in the neutral position. The physical examination should begin with a standard cardiopulmonary evaluation (airway, breathing, circulation).

Airway compromise may occur as a result of obstruction or neuromuscular dysfunction. Increased dependency on abdominal muscles for respiration (diaphragmatic breathing) caused by paralysis of the intercostal muscles may result from a spinal cord injury. An athlete may demonstrate signs of neurogenic shock (hypotension with bradycardia).

If the athlete is breathing and has a pulse, the mouth guard should be removed and the airway maintained. Remove the face mask only if the respiratory status is compromised. The helmet and chin strap should be left in place. The sagittal alignment of the cervical spine in football players wearing shoulder pads most closely approximates normal when the helmet remains in place.[107] The level of consciousness, response to pain, pupillary response, and any unusual posturing, flaccidity, rigidity, or weakness should be noted. The situation is maintained until transportation arrives. If the athlete is face-down, he or she may be log rolled onto the spine board when the ambulance arrives.

If the athlete is not breathing or stops breathing, the airway must be established. Prone athletes should be log rolled into the supine position, preferably onto a spine board. Log rolling ideally requires four individuals: three to roll and one person, the leader, to control the head and give commands.[133,134] A fifth member of the team is required to help lift and carry when necessary. The three assistants of the medical support team are positioned at the shoulders, hips, and knees, respectively (Fig. 9-15).

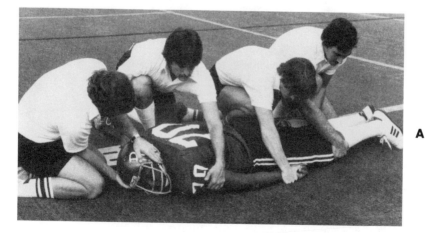

**Fig. 9-15.** Log roll onto a spine board. **A,** This maneuver requires four individuals: a leader to immobilize the head and neck and to command the medical support team, and three individuals who are positioned at the athlete's shoulders, hips, and knees. (With permission from Vegso JJ, Torg JS: Field evaluation and management of cervical spine injuries. In Torg JS: *Athletic injuries to the head, neck, and face,* ed 2, St Louis, 1991, Mosby–Year Book.)

*Continued*

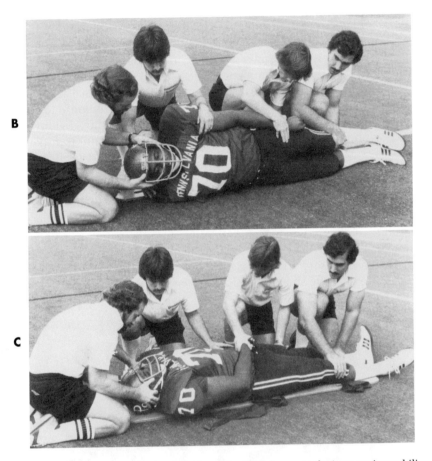

**Fig. 9-15, cont'd. B,** The leader uses the crossed-arm technique to immobilize the head. This technique allows the leader's arms to "unwind" as the three assistants roll the athlete onto the spine board. **C,** The three assistants maintain body alignment during the roll. (With permission from Vegso JJ, Torg JS: Field evaluation and management of cervical spine injuries. In Torg JS: *Athletic injuries to the head, neck, and face,* ed 2, St Louis, 1991, Mosby–Year Book.)

*Continued*

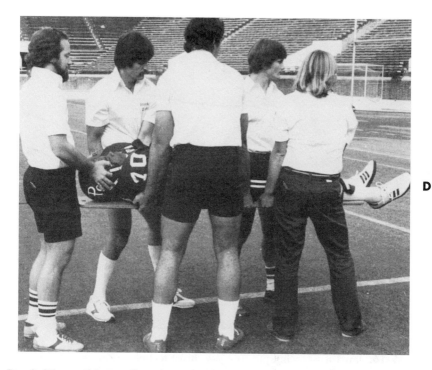

**D**

**Fig. 9-15, cont'd. D,** Lift and carry requires a fifth member of the team. Four members of the medical support team lift the athlete on the command of the leader. The leader maintains manual immobilization of the head.

The athlete is carefully rolled toward the assistants. The athlete's body is maintained in line with the head and spine during the maneuver. The leader maintains immobilization of the head by applying slight traction and by using the crossed-arm technique.

Once the athlete is supine, the face mask must be removed. The athlete's respiratory and circulatory status should be reassessed. If there is no breathing or if breathing has stopped, the airway must be established. The jaw thrust technique should be utilized to establish the airway. The jaw thrust technique is the safest first approach to opening the airway of a victim who is suspected of having neck injury.[22] The technique requires grasping the angles of the victim's lower jaw and lifting with both hands (one on each side), thereby displacing the mandible forward while tilting the head backward. The rescuer's elbows should rest on the surface on which the victim is lying (Fig. 9-16).

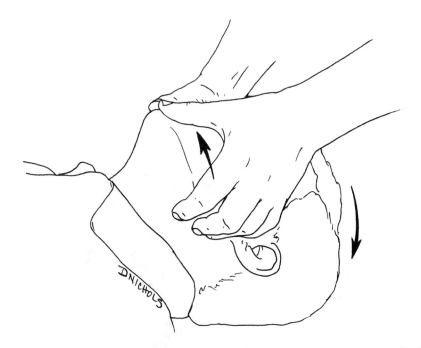

**Fig. 9-16.** Jaw thrust technique. The jaw thrust technique can be accomplished by grasping the angles of the victim's lower jaw and lifting with both hands (one on each side), thereby placing the mandible forward while tilting the head backward. The rescuer's elbows should rest on the surface on which the victim is lying.

If the jaw thrust maneuver is inadequate, the head tilt–jaw lift technique should be used.[22] One hand is placed on the victim's forehead and firm, backward pressure is applied with the palm to tilt the head back. The fingers of the other hand are placed under the bony part of the lower jaw near the chin and lifted to bring the chin forward and the teeth almost to occlusion, thus supporting the jaw and helping tilt the head back (Fig. 9-17). The fingers must not compress the soft tissue under the chin, which might obstruct the airway. Prompt resuscitation should proceed according to guidelines established by the American Heart Association.[22]

Once the athlete has arrived at the proper medical facility, the helmet may be removed. The chin strap and cheek pads are removed. The athlete's head is supported at the occiput while the leader spreads the earflaps and pulls the helmet off in a straight line with the spine (Fig. 9-18).

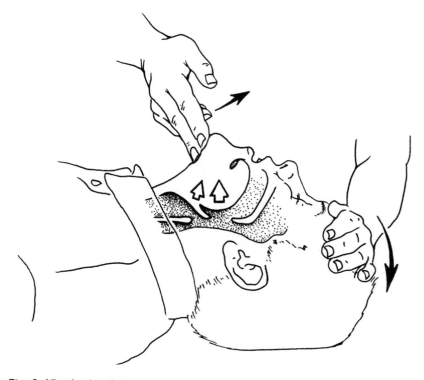

**Fig. 9-17.** The head tilt–jaw lift technique. One hand is placed on the victim's forehead, and firm backward pressure is applied with the palm to tilt the head back. The fingers of the other hand are placed under the bony part of the lower jaw near the chin and lifted to bring the chin forward and the teeth almost to occlusion, thus supporting the jaw and helping tilt the head back.

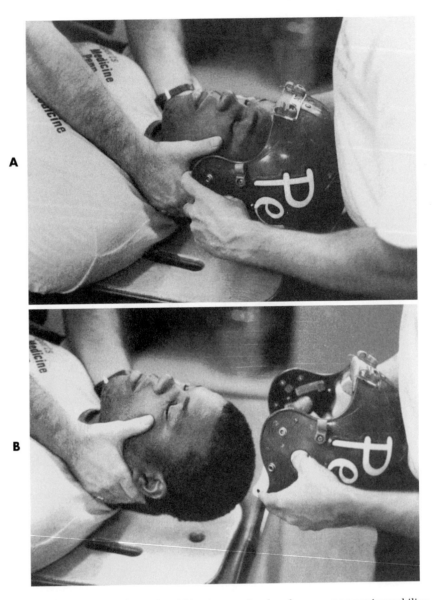

**Fig. 9-18. A,** The helmet should be removed only when permanent immobilization can be instituted. The helmet may be removed by detaching the chin strap, spreading the earflaps, and gently pulling the helmet off in a straight line with the cervical spine. **B,** The head must be supported under the occiput during and after removing the helmet. (With permission from Vegso JJ, Torg JS: Field evaluation and management of cervical spine injuries. In Torg JS: *Athletic injuries to the head, neck, and face,* ed 2, St Louis, 1991, Mosby–Year Book.)

# RETURN-TO-PLAY CRITERIA

Athletes who sustain cervical spine sprains and strains may return to contact sports if clinical examination yields these findings: (1) full, painless cervical spine range of motion, (2) no weakness, and (3) a normal neurologic evaluation. The presence of neck pain, weakness, or sensory changes should raise concern about the possibility of a cervical spine fracture or more serious injury.

Torg and colleagues[117,118] have recently established criteria for return to contact sports for a variety of bony and ligamentous injury patterns. Six major injury categories have been identified: (1) congenital, (2) developmental, (3) traumatic injury of the upper cervical spine (C1 to C2), (4) traumatic injury to the middle (C3 to C4) and lower (C5 to C7) cervical spine, (5) intervertebral disk injury, and (6) status postcervical spine fusion. Each specific condition has been determined to present either no contraindication, a relative contraindication, or an absolute contraindication to return to contact sports.

## NO CONTRAINDICATION

Spina bifida occulta—a rare, congenital anomaly—presents no contraindication to return to contact sports. A type II Klippel-Feil anomaly (fusion of only one or two interspaces) in an asymptomatic patient with a full range of cervical spine motion; no cervicooccipital anomalies; and no instability, disk disease, or degenerative changes presents no contraindication to return to contact sports. Asymptomatic individuals with cervical stenosis (Torg ratio less than 0.8), stable one-level anterior or posterior fusions, and healed anterior or lateral disk herniations treated conservatively represent no contraindications to return to contact sports. Clay shoveler's fractures, stable compression fractures, and end plate fractures without sagittal components or posterior ligamentous instability also represent no contraindications to return to contact sports.

## RELATIVE CONTRAINDICATION

Healed, nondisplaced Jefferson's fractures; healed type I and type II odontoid fractures; and healed lateral mass fractures of C2 in patients with full, pain-free cervical spine range of motion and normal neurologic examination represent relative contraindications to return to contact sports. Asymptomatic athletes with stable two- or three-level fusions and healed, displaced body fractures with no sagittal component present relative contraindications to return to contact sports. Individuals with cervical stenosis (Torg ratio less than 0.8) who sustain a documented episode of transient quadriplegia, and athletes with herniated disks treated conservatively or with surgery with residual facet instability also represent a relative contraindication to return to contact sports. Finally, any stable ligamentous injury in the middle or lower cervical spine (less than 3.5 mm translation or less than 11 degrees angulation) presents a relative contraindication to return to contact sports.

## ABSOLUTE CONTRAINDICATION

The presence of any congenital odontoid abnormality—including os odontoideum, odontoid agenesis, or odontoid hypoplasia—represents an absolute contraindication to return to contact sports. Athletes with congenital atlantooccipital fusions; type I Klippel-Feil syndrome (mass fusion); symptomatic type II Klippel-Feil syndrome; spear tackler's spine; fusions involving C1 or C2; or fusions extending beyond four or more levels should not participate in contact sports. Acute fractures of the vertebral body or posterior elements, as well as acute central disk herniations, represent absolute contraindications to return to contact sports. Acute or chronic "hard disk" herniations with associated neurologic findings, as well as pain or limitation of motion or those associated with cord neurapraxia resulting from concomitant cervical stenosis, represent absolute contraindications to return to contact sports. Likewise, the following healed fractures preclude further participation in contact sports:

1. Lateral mass fracture with facet incongruity
2. Displaced vertebral body fracture with a sagittal component
3. Fracture of C1 or C2 with ligamentous instability
4. Vertebral body fracture with ligamentous instability or an associated posterior arch fracture
5. Comminuted body fracture with displacement into the cervical canal
6. Vertebral body or posterior element fracture with pain, neurologic findings, or decreased cervical range of motion
7. Any lesion with MRI evidence of a cord defect or swelling

Individuals demonstrating instability in the middle or lower cervical spine (greater than 3.5 mm translation or greater than 11 degrees angulation) should also be restricted from contact sports. Finally, any athlete with cervical stenosis (Torg ratio less than 0.8) who experiences a documented episode of transient quadriplegia in association with ligamentous instability, disk disease, degenerative changes, MRI evidence of a cord defect or swelling, neurologic deficits lasting beyond 36 hours, or more than one recurrence should not continue to participate in contact sports.

## SUMMARY

Athletic injuries to the cervical spine are not uncommon. Fortunately, most injuries do not result in permanent disability. Prior planning is necessary to avoid potential catastrophic sequelae. Criteria have been established to determine whether an athlete may or may not return to contact sports. Axial loading is the principal mechanism responsible for most serious athletic cervical spine injuries. Prompt recognition, appropriate assessment, and proper treatment are essential for the safe and timely return of the injured athlete to participation.

## References

1. Adelstein W, Watson P: Cervical spine injuries, *J Neurosurg Nurs* 15:65-71, 1983.
2. Albrand OW, Corkill G: Broken necks from diving accidents: a summer epidemic in young men, *Am J Sports Med* 4:107-110, 1976.
3. Albrand OW, Walter J: Underwater deceleration curves in relation to injuries from diving, *Surg Neurol* 4:461-465, 1975.
4. Albright JP, McAuley E, Martin RK et al: Head and neck injuries in college football: an eight-year analysis, *Am J Sports Med* 13:147-152, 1985.
5. Albright JP, Moses JM, Feldick HG et al: Nonfatal cervical spine injuries in interscholastic football, *JAMA* 236:1243-1245, 1976.
6. Alem NM, Nusholtz GS, Melvin JW: Head and neck response to axial impacts. Proceedings of the twenty-eighth Stapp Car Crash Conference, Society of Automotive Engineers, Warrendale, Pa, 1984.
7. Allen BL Jr, Ferguson RL, Lehman TR et al: A mechanistic classification of closed indirect fractures and dislocations of the lower cervical spine, *Spine* 7:1-27, 1982.
8. Allen RL, Perot PL Jr, Gudeman SK: Evaluation of acute nonpenetrating cervical spinal cord injuries with CT metrizamide myelography, *J Neurosurg* 63:510-520, 1985.
9. Anderson LD, D'Alonzo RT: Fractures of the odontoid process of the axis, *J Bone Joint Surg* 56A:663-674, 1974.
10. Andrish JT, Bergfeld JA, Romo L: A method for the management of cervical injuries in football: a preliminary report, *Am J Sports Med* 5:89-92, 1977.
11. Apple DF Jr, McDonald AP, Smith RA: Identification of herniated nucleus pulposus in spinal cord injury, *Paraplegia* 25:78-85, 1987.
12. Apuzzo MLJ, Heiden JS, Weiss MH et al: Acute fractures of the odontoid process: an analysis of 45 cases, *J Neurosurg* 48:85-91, 1978.
13. Bauze RJ, Ardran GM: Experimental production of forward dislocation in the human cervical spine, *J Bone Joint Surg* 60B:239-245, 1978.
14. Bishop PJ, Wells RP: Cervical spine fractures: mechanisms, neck loads, and methods of prevention. In Castaldi CR, Hoerner ER, editors: *Safety in ice hockey*, Philadelphia, 1989, American Society for Testing and Materials.
15. Bohlman HH, Davis DD: The pathology of fatal craniospinal injuries. In Brinkhous KM, editor: *Accident pathology: proceedings of an international conference*, Washington, DC, 1970, US Government Printing Office.
16. Bracken MB, Shepard MJ, Collins WF et al: A randomized controlled trial of methylprednisolone or naloxone in the treatment of acute spinal-cord injury: results of the second national acute spinal cord injury study, *N Engl J Med* 322:1405-1411, 1990.
17. Brooke WS: Complete transverse cervical myelitis caused by traumatic herniation of an ossified nucleus pulposus, *JAMA* 125:117-120, 1944.
18. Cantu RC: Catastrophic injuries of high school and collegiate athletes, *Surg Rounds Orthop* 2:62-66, 1988.
19. Cantu RC, Mueller FO: Catastrophic spine injuries in football (1977-1989), *J Spinal Disord* 3:227-231, 1990.

20. Carter DR, Frankel VH: Biomechanics of hyperextension injuries of the cervical spine in football, *Am J Sports Med* 8:302-308, 1980.
21. Carvell JE, Fuller DJ, Duthrie RB et al: Rugby football injuries to the cervical spine, *BMJ* 286:49-50, 1983.
22. Chandra NC, Hazinski MF, editors: *Textbook of basic life support for healthcare providers*, Dallas, 1994, American Heart Association.
23. Clark CR, White AA: Fractures of the dens: a multicenter study, *J Bone Joint Surg* 67A:1340-1348, 1985.
24. Clark KS: An epidemiologic view. In Torg JS, editor: *Athletic injuries to the head, neck, and face*, Philadelphia, 1982, Lea & Febiger.
25. Cloward RB: Acute cervical spine injuries, *Clin Symp* 32:2-32, 1980.
26. Coin CG, Pennink M, Ahmad WD et al: Diving-type injury of the cervical spine: contribution of computed tomography to management, *J Comput Assist Tomogr* 3:362-372, 1979.
27. Dall DM: Injuries of the cervical spine, *S Afr Med J* 46:1048-1056, 1972.
28. Davis D, Bohlman H, Walker AE et al: The pathological findings in fatal craniospinal injuries, *J Neurosurg* 34:603-613, 1971.
29. De Oliveira JC: Anterior reduction of interlocking facets in the lower cervical spine, *Spine* 4:195-202, 1979.
30. Dolan KD, Feldick HG, Albright JP et al: Neck injuries in football players, *Am Fam Physician* 12:86-91, 1975.
31. Dorwart R, LeMasters DL: Application of computed tomographic scanning of the cervical spine, *Orthop Clin North Am* 16:381-393, 1985.
32. Durbin FC: Fracture-dislocations of the cervical spine, *J Bone Joint Surg* 39B:23-38, 1957.
33. Eismont FJ, Arena MJ, Green BA: Extrusion of an intravertebral disc associated with traumatic subluxation or dislocation of cervical facets, *J Bone Joint Surg* 73A:1555-1560, 1991.
34. Ellis WG, Green D, Holzaepfel NR et al: The trampoline and serious neurological injuries: a report of five cases, *JAMA* 174:1673-1677, 1960.
35. Esses S: Fracture of the atlas associated with fracture of the odontoid process, *Injury* 12:310-312, 1981.
36. Evans RF: Tetraplegia caused by gymnastics, *BMJ* 2:732, 1979.
37. Fielding JW, Cochran GVB, Lawsing JF et al: Tears of the transverse ligament of the atlas: a clinical and biomechanical study, *J Bone Joint Surg* 56A:1683-1691, 1974.
38. Fielding WJ, Stillwell WT, Chynn KY et al: Use of computed tomography for the diagnosis of atlanto-axial rotatory fixation, *J Bone Joint Surg* 60A:1102-1104, 1978.
39. Frykman G, Hilding S: Hop pa studsmatta kan orska allvarliga skador (Trampoline jumping can cause serious injury). *Lakartidningen* 67:5862-5864, 1970.
40. Funk FJ Jr, Wells RE: Injuries of the cervical spine in football, *Clin Orthop* 109:50-58, 1975.
41. Garger WN, Fisher RG, Halfmann HW: Vertebrectomy and fusion for "teardrop fracture" of the cervical spine: case report, *J Trauma* 9:887-893, 1969.
42. Gehweiler JH, Clark WM, Schaaf R et al: Cervical spine trauma: the common combined conditions, *Radiology* 130:77-86, 1979.
43. Gosch HH, Gooding E, Schneider RC: An experimental study of cervical spine and cord injuries, *J Trauma* 12:570-576, 1972.
44. Griffin LY, editor: *Orthopaedic knowledge update: sports medicine*, Rosemont, Ill, 1994, American Academy of Orthopaedic Surgeons.
45. Grogono BJS: Injuries of the atlas and axis, *J Bone Joint Surg* 36B:397-410, 1954.
46. Haines JD: Occult cervical spine fractures, *Postgrad Med* 80:73-77, 1986.

47. Hammer A, Schwartzbach AL, Darre E et al: Svaere neurologiske skader some folge af trampolinspring (Severe neurologic damage resulting from trampolining), *Ugeskrift Laeger* 143:2970-2974, 1981.
48. Herrick RT: Clay shovelers' fracture in power lifting: a case report, *Am J Sports Med* 9:29-30, 1981.
49. Herzog RJ, Wiens JJ, Dillingham MF et al: Normal cervical spine morphometry and cervical spinal stenosis in asymptomatic professional football players, *Spine* 16(suppl 6):S178-S186, 1991.
50. Hinck VC, Hopkins CE, Savara BS: Sagittal diameter of the cervical spinal canal in children, *Radiology* 79:97-108, 1962.
51. Hodgson VR, Thomas LM: Mechanisms of cervical spine injury during impact to the protected head. Proceedings of the twenty-fourth Stapp Car Crash Conference, 1980.
52. Jackson DW, Lohr FT: Cervical spine injuries, *Clin Sports Med* 5:373-386, 1986.
53. Jefferson G: Fracture of the atlas vertebra: report of four cases and review of those previously recorded, *Br J Surg* 7:47-422, 1920.
54. Kazarian L: Injuries to the human spinal column: biomechanics and injury classification, *Exerc Sports Sci Rev* 9:297-352, 1981.
55. Kewalramani LS, Taylor RG: Injuries to the cervical spine from diving accidents, *J Trauma* 15:130-142, 1975.
56. King DM: Fractures and dislocations of the cervical spine, *Austral N Z J Surg* 37:57-64, 1967
57. Leidholt JD: Spinal injuries in athletes: be prepared, *Orthop Clin North Am* 4:691-707, 1973.
58. Levine AM, Edwards C: The management of traumatic spondylolisthesis of the axis, *J Bone Joint Surg* 67A:217-226, 1985.
59. Levine AM, Edwards C: Treatment of injuries in the C1-C2 complex, *Orthop Clin North Am* 17:31-44, 1986.
60. MacNab I: Acceleration injuries of the cervical spine, *J Bone Joint Surg* 46A:1797-1799, 1964.
61. Maiman DJ, Sances A, Myklebust JB et al: Compression injuries of the cervical spine: a biomechanical analysis, *Neurosurgery* 13:254-260, 1983.
62. Marks MR, Bell GR, Boumphrey FR: Cervical spine fractures in athletes, *Clin Sports Med* 9:13-29, 1990.
63. Maroon JC, Steele PB, Berlin R: Football head and neck injuries: an update, *Clin Neurosurg* 27:414-429, 1979.
64. McCoy GF, Piggot J, Macafee AL et al: Injuries of the cervical spine in schoolboy rugby football, *J Bone Joint Surg* 66B:500-503, 1984.
65. Mennen U: Survey of spinal injuries from diving: a study of patients in Pretoria and Cape Town, *S Afr Med J* 59:788-790, May 1981.
66. Mertz HJ, Hodgson VR, Murray TL et al: An assessment of compressive neck loads under injury-producing conditions, *Physician Sports Med* 6:95-106, 1978.
67. Meyer SA, Schulte KR, Callaghan JJ et al: Cervical spinal stenosis and stingers in collegiate football players, *Am J Sports Med* 22:158-166, 1994.
68. Mueller FO, Blyth CS: Fatalities from head and cervical spine injuries occurring in tackle football: 40 years' experience, *Clin Sports Med* 6:185-196, 1987.
69. Mueller FO, Cantu RC: Catastrophic injuries and fatalities in high school and college sports, fall 1982-spring 1988, *Med Sci Sports Exerc* 22:737-741, 1990.
70. Norrell HA: Fractures and dislocations of the spine. In Rothman RH, Simeone FA, editors: *The spine*, vol 2, Philadelphia, 1975, WB Saunders.
71. Nuber GW, Schafer MF: Clay shovelers' injuries: a report of two injuries sustained from football, *Am J Sports Med* 15:182-183, 1987.

72. O'Carroll F, Sheenan M, Gregg TM: Cervical spine injuries in rugby football, *Ir Med J* 74:377-379, 1981.

73. Odor JM, Watkins RG, Dillin WH et al: Incidence of cervical spinal stenosis in professional and rookie football players, *Am J Sports Med* 18:507-509, 1990.

74. Otis JC, Burstein AH, Torg JS: Mechanisms and pathomechanics of athletic injuries to the cervical spine. In Torg JS, editor, *Athletic injuries to the head, neck, and face*, ed 2, Philadelphia, 1991, Mosby–Year Book.

75. Paley D, Gillespie R: Chronic repetitive unrecognized flexion injury of the cervical spine (high jumpers neck), *Am J Sports Med* 14:92-95, 1986.

76. Petrie JG: Flexion injuries of the cervical spine, *J Bone Joint Surg* 46A:1800-1806, 1964.

77. Piggot J, Gordon DS: Rugby injuries to the cervical cord, *BMJ* 1:192-193, 1979.

78. Powers B, Miller MD, Kramer RS et al: Traumatic atlanto-occipital dislocation with survival, *Neurosurgery* 4:12-17, 1979.

79. Raynor RB: Cervical cord compression secondary to acute disk protrusion in trauma: incidence and response to decompression, *Spine* 2:39-43, 1977.

80. Reynen PD, Clancy WG Jr: Cervical spine injury, hockey helmets, and face masks, *Am J Sports Med* 22:167-170, 1994.

81. Richman S, Friedman R: Vertical fracture of cervical vertebral bodies, *Radiology* 62:536-542, 1954.

82. Roaf R: A study of the mechanics of spinal injuries, *J Bone Joint Surg* 42B:810-823, 1960.

83. Rogers WA: Fractures and dislocations of the cervical spine: an end-result study, *J Bone Joint Surg* 39A:341-376, 1957.

84. Ruflin G, Jeanneret B, Magerl F: Tetraplegia following cervical spine fusion. Paper presented at the annual meeting of the Cervical Spine Research Society—European section, St Gallen, Switzerland, June 27, 1989.

85. Sances AJ, Myklebust JB, Maiman DJ et al: Biomechanics of spinal injuries, *Crit Rev Biomed Eng* 11:1-76, 1984.

86. Scher AT: Cervical vertebral dislocation in a rugby player with congenital vertebral fusion, *Br J Sports Med* 24:167-168, 1990.

87. Scher AT: "Crashing" the rugby scrum: an avoidable cause of cervical spinal injury, *S Afr Med J* 61:919-920, 1982.

88. Scher AT: Diving injuries to the cervical spinal cord, *S Afr Med J* 59:603-605, 1981.

89. Scher AT: Radiographic indicators of traumatic cervical spine instability, *S Afr Med J* 62:562-565, 1982.

90. Scher AT: Rugby injuries of the spine and spinal cord, *Clin Sports Med* 6:87-99, 1987.

91. Scher AT: "Teardrop" fractures of the cervical spine: radiologic features, *S Afr Med J* 61:355-359, 1982.

92. Scher AT: The high rugby tackle: an avoidable cause of cervical spinal injury? *S Afr Med J* 53:1015-1018, 1978.

93. Scher AT: Vertex impact and cervical dislocation in rugby players, *S Afr Med J* 59:227-228, 1981.

94. Schneider RC: *Head and neck injuries in football*, Baltimore, 1973, Williams & Wilkins.

95. Schneider RC: Serious and fatal neurosurgical football injuries, *Clin Neurosurg* 12:226-236, 1966.

96. Schneider RC: The syndrome of acute anterior spinal cord injury, *J Neurosurg* 12:95-123, 1955.

97. Schneider RC, Kahn EA: Chronic neurological sequelae of acute trauma to the spine and spinal cord. Part I. The significance of the acute-flexion or "tear-drop" fracture dislocation of the cervical spine, *J Bone Joint Surg* 38A:985-987, 1956.

98. Segal LS, Grimm JO, Stauffer ES: Non-union of fractures of the atlas, *J Bone Joint Surg* 69A:1423-1434, 1987.

99. Silver JR: Injuries of the spine sustained in rugby, *BMJ* 288:37-43, 1984.
100. Silver JR: Spinal injuries in sports in the UK, *Br J Sports Med* 27:115-120, 1993.
101. Silver JR, Silver DD, Godfrey JJ: Injuries of the spine sustained during gymnastic activities, *BMJ* 293:861-863, 1986.
102. Sim FH, Chao EY: Injury potential in modern ice hockey, *Am J Sports Med* 6:378-384, 1978.
103. Spence KF, Decker S, Sell KW: Bursting atlantal fracture associated with rupture of the transverse ligament, *J Bone Joint Surg* 52A:543-549, 1970.
104. Stauffer ES, Kaufer H: Fractures and dislocations of the spine. In Rockwood CA Jr, Green DP, editors: *Fractures*, vol 2, Philadelphia, 1975, JB Lippincott.
105. Steel HH: Anatomical and mechanical considerations of the atlanto-axial articulations: proceedings of the AOA. *J Bone Joint Surg* 50A:1481-1482, 1968.
106. Steinbruck J, Paeslack V: Trampolinspringen-ein gefahrlicher sport? (Is trampolining a dangerous sport?) *Munchener Medizinischer Wochenschrift* 120:985-988, 1978.
107. Swenson TM, Lauerman WC, Donaldson WF et al: Cervical spine alignment in the immobilized football player: radiographic analysis before and after helmet removal. Paper presented at the sixty-second annual meeting of the American Academy of Orthopaedic Surgery, Orlando, 1995.
108. Tator CH: Neck injuries in ice hockey: a recent unsolved problem with many contributing factors, *Clin Sports Med* 6:101-114, 1987.
109. Tator CH, Edmonds VE: National survey of spinal injuries in hockey players, *Can Med Assoc J* 130:875-880, 1984.
110. Tator CH, Edmonds VE, Lapczak L et al: Spinal injuries in ice hockey players 1966-1987, *Can J Surg* 34:63-69, 1991.
111. Tator CH, Edmonds VE, New ML: Diving: frequent and potentially preventable cause of spinal cord injury, *Can Med Assoc J* 124:1323-1324, 1982.
112. Tator CH, Ekong CE, Rowed DW et al: Spinal injuries due to hockey, *Can J Neurol Sci* 11:34-41, 1984.
113. Torg JS: Cervical spinal stenosis with cord neurapraxia and transient quadriplegia, *Clin Sports Med* 9:279-296, 1990.
114. Torg JS: Management guidelines for athletic injuries to the cervical spine, *Clin Sports Med* 6:53-60, 1987.
115. Torg JS: Trampoline-induced quadriplegia, *Clin Sports Med* 6:73-85, 1987.
116. Torg JS, Das M: Trampoline-related quadriplegia: review of the literature and reflections on the American Academy of Pediatrics' position statement, *Pediatrics* 74:804-812, 1984.
117. Torg JS, Glasgow SG: Criteria for return to contact activities after cervical spine injury. In Torg JS, editor: *Athletic injuries to the head, neck, and face*, ed 2, Philadelphia, 1991, Mosby–Year Book.
118. Torg JS, Glasgow SG: Criteria for return to contact activities following cervical spine injury, *Clin J Sports Med* 1:12-26, 1991.
119. Torg JS, Pavlov H: Cervical spinal stenosis with cord neurapraxia and transient quadriplegia, *Clin Sport Med* 6:115-133, 1987.
120. Torg JS, Pavlov H, Genuario SE et al: Neurapraxia of the cervical spinal cord with transient quadriplegia, *J Bone Joint Surg* 68A:1354-1370, 1988.
121. Torg JS, Pavlov H, O'Neill MJ et al: The axial load teardrop fracture. A biomechanical, clinical, and roentgenographic analysis, *Am J Sports Med* 19:355-364, 1991.
122. Torg JS, Quedenfeld TC, Burstein A et al: National football head and neck injury registry: report on cervical quadriplegia, 1971-1975, *Am J Sports Med* 7:127-132, 1979.
123. Torg JS, Quedenfeld TC, Moyer RA et al: Severe and catastrophic neck injuries resulting from tackle football, *J Am Coll Health Assoc* 25:224-266, 1977.

124. Torg JS, Sennett B, Pavlov H et al: Spear tackler's spine. An entity precluding participation in tackle football and collision activities that expose the cervical spine to axial energy inputs, *Am J Sports Med* 21:640-649, 1993.

125. Torg JS, Sennett B, Vegso JJ: Spinal injury at the level of the third and fourth cervical vertebrae resulting from the axial loading mechanism: An analysis and classification, *Clin Sports Med* 6:159-183, 1987.

126. Torg JS, Sennett B, Vegso JJ et al: Axial loading injuries to the middle cervical spine segment. An analysis and classification of 25 cases, *Am J Sports Med* 19:6-20, 1991.

127. Torg JS, Truex RC, Marshall J et al: Spinal injury at the level of the third and fourth cervical vertebrae from football, *J Bone Joint Surg* 59A:1015-1019, 1977.

128. Torg JS, Truex R Jr, Quedenfeld TC et al: National football head and neck injury registry: report and conclusions (1978), *JAMA* 241:1477-1479, 1979.

129. Torg JS, Vegso JJ, O'Neill MJ et al: The epidemiologic, pathologic, biomechanical, cinematographic analysis of football-induced cervical spine trauma, *Am J Sports Med* 18:50-57, 1990.

130. Torg JS, Vegso JJ, Sennett B: The national football head and neck injury registry: 14-year report on cervical quadriplegia (1971-1984), *Clin Sports Med* 6:61-72, 1987.

131. Torg JS, Vegso JJ, Sennett B et al: The national football head and neck injury registry. 14-year report on cervical quadriplegia (1971-1984), *JAMA* 254:3439-3443, 1985.

132. Torg JS, Wiesel SW, Rothman RH: Diagnosis and management of cervical spine injuries. In Torg JS, editor: *Athletic injuries to the head, neck, and face,* Philadelphia, 1982, Lea & Febiger.

133. Vegso JJ, Lehman RC: Field evaluation and management of head and neck injuries, *Clin Sports Med* 6:1-15, 1987.

134. Vegso JJ, Torg JS: Field evaluation and management of cervical spine injuries. In Torg JS, editor: *Athletic injuries to the head, neck, and face,* ed 2, Philadelphia, 1991, Mosby–Year Book.

135. Virgin H: Cineradiographic study of football helmets and the cervical spine, *Am J Sports Med* 8:310-317, 1980.

136. Von Torklus D, Gehle W: *The upper cervical spine,* New York, 1972, Grune & Stratton.

137. Watkins RG: Neck injuries in football players, *Clin Sports Med* 5:215-246, 1986.

138. White AA III, Panjabi MM: *Clinical biomechanics of the spine,* ed 2, Philadelphia, 1990, JB Lippincott.

139. White AA III, Johnson RM, Panjabi MM et al: Biomechanical analysis of clinical stability in the cervical spine, *Clin Orthop* 109:85-96, 1975.

140. Whitley JE, Forsyth HF: The classification of cervical spine injuries, *Am J Roentgenol* 83:633-644, 1960.

141. Williams JPR, McKibbin B: Cervical spine injuries in rugby union football, *BMJ* 2:1747, 1978.

142. Williams P, McKibbin B: Unstable cervical spine injuries in rugby: a 20 year review, *Injury* 18:329-332, 1987.

143. Wu WQ, Lewis RC: Injuries of the cervical spine in high school wrestling, *Surg Neurol* 23:143-147, 1985.

# CHAPTER 10

# Injuries to the low back

J. Stanford Faulkner, Jr.
J. Markus Carter
Scott Deuel

Injuries to the low back are relatively common among athletes. However, little attention is usually given to this subject since it is not a "hot topic" in sports medicine circles. Many studies have shown varying rates of low back injuries in different sports. Studies have shown that up to 30% of college football players and 12% of NFL players have lost time playing as a result of low back injuries; in professional basketball, low back injuries usually rank third in occurrence behind ankle and knee injuries. Previous surveys of French ballet dancers have revealed a 25% frequency of spine injuries in males and 20% in females. A study by Glick and Katch in 1970 found that about 9% of middle-aged joggers had complaints of low back pain. Other studies have shown the incidence of these injuries among gymnasts to be up to 79%. These low back injuries can vary from fractures to soft tissue injuries. Just as with injuries to the extremities, most of these low back problems can be acutely treated on the field. If given an accurate diagnosis, appropriate management on the field, and efficient rehabilitation, the athelete can be expediently and safely returned to play by the treating sports medicine personnel.

## INITIAL ASSESSMENT

The most important component, when initially assessing a player for a low back injury, should be the ruling out of possible neurologic involvement. Injured muscles, bones, tendons, and ligaments usually recover and leave the patient asymptomatic. Spinal cord or nerve injury can be permanent and can have a devastating sequela, such as paralysis, numbness, weakness, loss of bowel or bladder control, or chronic pain. Although neurologic injury comprises 1% or less of all athletic injuries, it should be ruled out first. Obvious signs of neurologic involvement include weakness of the lower extremities, numbness, loss of bowel or bladder control, or pain radiating into the legs. If these neurologic symptoms are present and persist, the patient should be transported for medical attention.

Objective information for neurologic involvement should also be obtained immediately. This includes any notable weakness that can be checked by having the athlete dorsiflex and plantarflex both feet and flex and extend both hips and knees. A brief sensory check includes having the player respond to light touch on the lateral and medial aspects of the feet and legs. Any obvious signs of bowel or bladder incontinence would suggest a medical emergency. Once neurologic involvement has been ruled out, further assessment of the injury should follow.

Back pain is the most prevalent complaint of injuries to the low back. The cause of this pain is often difficult to determine. Initial assessments should include determining the mechanism of the injury. Was there a direct blow? Was there axial loading with either flexion or extension? Was there a rotational injury? Or was there a combination of all of these mechanisms? The acuteness of the pain should be evaluated to determine whether the cause was one single incident or the result of repetitive trauma. The nature, location, and severity of the pain should be elicited, as well as any radiation of the pain. Localizing the pain and determining the mechanism of injury can lead to the cause of the pain. A direct blow will cause a bruise or contusion with possible swelling or redness.

After obtaining the history of the mechanism of the injury and the location and nature of the complaint, a physical exam or objective assessment should be performed. On gross assessment, attention should be paid to the pain behaviors, obvious deformities, postural deviation, or color changes that are signs of contusions or abrasions. Palpation of the involved area should be performed with notation of tenderness, edema, muscle spasm, or any defects or deformities. Range of motion should then be assessed, noting any changes in pain and any muscle guarding. Again, a neurologic assessment is also done during this portion of the evaluation. This includes a brief sensory and motor exam, as has been mentioned previously in this chapter. A check for light touch sensation on the lower extremities should be done, and the athlete should flex and extend the hips, knees, and ankles for a quick assessment of motor function.

The aforementioned evaluation can be done on the field. If the severity of the complaints is such that the athlete is experiencing neurologic symptoms or is otherwise functionally impaired, then further medical evaluation must be pursued immediately. Use of a spine board for immobilization provides the safest immediate transportation to a medical facility for further evaluation.

## DIFFERENTIAL DIAGNOSIS

Most often the final diagnosis for a low back injury is a diagnosis of exclusion. This is the case when most of the objective tests performed—such as x-rays, magnetic resonance imaging (MRI), and computed tomography (CT) scans—are normal. Many different terms and diagnoses are assigned to low back pain.

Lumbar sprains most commonly occur from hyperflexion, hyperextension, excessive rotation, and excessive side-bending of the lumbar spine. Hyperflexion can result in a sprain of several ligaments, including supraspinous, interspinous, iliolumbar, and posterior longitudinal ligaments. Lumbar sprains are diagnosed with injuries occurring to the lumbar musculature. Most sprains are a result of high intensity contractions from acceleration or deceleration forces on the lumbar spine; that is, "It wasn't the fall that killed him, it was the sudden stop."

Disk injury is thought to result from a combination of flexion, rotation, and compression. The earliest injury is believed to be an annular test, a slight break in the outer fibrous ring. This can lead to acute back pain and inflammation, with radicular pain into the affected lower extremity. If further breakdown occurs, herniation of the nucleus pulposus (i.e., a herniated disk) can occur. This can cause nerve root compression, which in turn produces symptoms such as pain, numbness, and weakness in the extremity. Valsalva's maneuver (such as coughing, sneezing, or bowel movement straining) may also reproduce leg pain. This type of injury is most often diagnosed through the use of MRI or CT scan.

Facet joint injury is often considered to result from extension and rotation forces, but it can also result from hyperflexion and compression. Since the facet joint is a synovial joint, it can become inflamed with swelling of the capsule and irritation of the adjacent nerves. Mechanical joint dysfunction is characterized by focal tenderness over a specific joint, with associated hyper- and hypomobility. Range of motion testing is usually asymmetrical. Joint dysfunction may accompany other conditions such as degenerative joint disease and diskogenic pathology.

Fractures in the lumbar spine that result from competitive sports are most commonly compression fractures of the vertebral body or stress fractures of the pars interarticularis. Compression fractures occur from axial loading of acute flexion. Pars fractures are often considered to result from repetitive hyperextension forces. Most of these pars defects are probably developmental defects but are aggravated by extension activities. Clinical correlation of lumbar spine x-rays and a bone scan is recommended for definitive diagnosis.

Degenerative disk and joint disease quite commonly accompanies aging; however, it can also be seen with overuse and repetitive trauma.

Symptoms associated with degenerative joint disease may be nonspecific in nature and are quite often associated with morning stiffness. Mechanical joint dysfunction, with associated frequent lumbar sprain and strain types of injuries, may often accompany degenerative joint disease.

Narrowing of the spinal canal (i.e., spinal stenosis) is either congenital or associated with degenerative joint disease, and it may cause low back pain or symptoms in the lower extremities. Acute or chronic compression of the spinal contents from spinal stenosis may cause symptoms of lower extremity claudication, such as tingling paresthesias and lower extremity weakness, especially after prolonged standing or walking. This must be distinguished from intermittent vascular claudication, which may have similar types of symptoms.

Spondylolisthesis, or the forward slipping of one vertebra over another or of the last lumbar vertebra over the sacrum, is seen quite commonly in athletes who engage in repetitive hyperextension maneuvers such as gymnastics and football. The forward slippage of the vertebra is caused by spondylolytic defect of the pars interarticularis. This defect may be secondary to trauma, bone disease, or congenital deformity. Spondylolisthesis is often asymptomatic until older adulthood; however, patients with symptomatic spondylolisthesis usually complain of low back pain that is often accompanied by sciatica.

Myofascial pain syndrome is characterized by regional muscular pain, with complaints of aching, soreness, and muscle stiffness. Characteristic points of muscular tenderness, known as "trigger points," are also associated with myofascial pain. On palpation these trigger points not only cause local tenderness at the spot of palpation, but also may radiate pain in a referred pattern over an entire muscle group. Myofascial pain syndromes are common sequelae to sprain-strain types of injuries. Myofascial pain also mimics symptoms of radiculopathy and diskogenic syndromes.

## TREATMENT

After the initial assessment, the treatment given to the injured athlete depends on the severity of injury, the amount of pain, and the impairment of the athlete's functional ability. The athlete's ability to return to play should be based on the athlete's degree of pain and his or her ability to perform athletic activities. Pain is the athlete's most common limitation. If the athlete has moderate to severe pain complaints, applying ice to the injured area can help decrease the pain and control any inflammation. Lumbar supports or braces can be beneficial to help control the athlete's symptoms. Braces are most effective after acute sprains, strains, or contusions. Flexibility exercises to help stretch the lumbar musculature and lower extremities often help control the athlete's symptoms and return the athlete to play. If the athlete is only experiencing minimal to moderate amounts of pain and can perform the athletic activities without experiencing pain, the decision to return the athlete to play is appropriate with the player and coach's consent.

Returning an athlete to play after a low back injury is most efficiently and safely performed with functional criteria. Ideally, before an athlete returns to play, the internal components—which can have a direct effect on the stress placed on the healing or healed tissues—should be addressed. These components include flexibility of the lower extremity—which encompasses the foot and ankle, up to and including the pelvis. Flexibility and strength of the lumbopelvic musculature should be normal. The athlete must also be able to demonstrate adequate neuromuscular control, which is basically the ability of the musculature to stabilize and control the low back. Regaining the neuromuscular control of the lumbopelvic region is as important as regaining proprioceptive awareness of the ankle after a sprain.

Once the internal criteria have been met, sports-specific training is the main focus. Breaking the sport into components allows for safe step-by-step return to play. For instance, a nose tackle must first perform exercises in the stance position correctly before any contact can be allowed. The next step could be manual resistance to the athlete in that stance, followed by exploding into the sled at one-quarter, half, three-quarters, to full effort. The final step would be full contact. Pain during the progression can be a limiting factor, and the amount of pain should be taken as a deterrent to further progression or return to play at that time.

Returning an athlete to competitive activities after a low back injury can be a very challenging task. The return of the athlete requires the team work of the athlete and the sports medicine personnel. With immediate medical intervention, diagnosis of the injury, and an organized and efficient treatment plan, the expedient and safe return of the athlete to play can be accomplished.

## Bibliography

Deyo RA, Dichl AK, Rosenthal M: How many days of bedrest for low back pain? *New Engl J Med* 315:1064-1070, 1986.

Ferguson RJ, McMaster JH, Stanitsk CL: Low back pain in college football linemen, *J Sports Med Phys Fitness* 2:63-69, 1974.

Morgan D: Concepts in functional training and postural stabilization for the low back injury, *Top Acute Care Trauma Rehabil,* pp 8-17, 1988.

Powell JW: Summary of injury patterns for seven seasons, 1980-1986. NFL Injury surveillance program, Department of Physical Education, San Diego University, San Diego, 1987.

Swaid L et al: Disc degeneration and associated abnormalities of the spine in elite gymnastics, *Spine* 16:437-443, 1991.

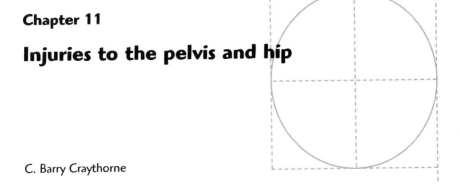

# Chapter 11

# Injuries to the pelvis and hip

C. Barry Craythorne

Injuries involving the pelvis and hip of an athlete may cause considerable disability. The ability to recognize and treat these injuries requires an understanding of the local anatomy, including bony, muscular, and ligamentous structures.

The hip joint is a ball-and-socket joint formed by the head of the femur and the acetabulum of the pelvis. The hip joint is inherently stable, not only because of its bony anatomic configuration, but also because of strong ligamentous support in the capsule of the joint. As a result, severe athletic injuries of the hip joint itself are rather rare.

The pelvis is an anatomically complex bony structure that functions to support the weight transmitted by the trunk and spine. Two paired iliac bones are joined posteriorly to the sacrum at the sacroiliac joints and anteriorly through the pubis at the symphysis pubis. Athletic injuries about the pelvis generally involve one of two mechanisms: (1) a direct contusion to soft tissues or bony prominences or (2) a musculotendinous strain involving any one of many muscular insertions about the pelvis.

## HIP POINTER

The hip pointer is considered the most disabling contusion of the pelvis and is common in contact sports. The anatomy of the region includes the iliac crest, to which the abdominal muscles attach from above and from which the gluteal muscles originate below. The iliac crest is the palpable bony prominence of the pelvis at the side of the body and is vulnerable to injury.

### MECHANISM OF INJURY

The hip pointer is a contusion of the iliac crest region. It usually results either from forceful contact in a fall to the ground or from a direct blow from an object such as a football helmet. A hematoma forms within the soft tissue at the point of contact along the iliac crest. This injury generally results from inadequate padding or protection of the iliac crest region.

## CLINICAL DIAGNOSIS

The athlete with a hip pointer will have difficulty running or walking normally because of pain and muscle spasm. Point tenderness is noted with palpation along the crest of the ilium. It may be noted that the player's hip padding is abnormally loose or positioned too low.

## DIFFERENTIAL DIAGNOSIS

Two other conditions should be considered in the differential diagnosis of a hip pointer. The first is an avulsion or fracture of the iliac apophysis, which is the area of growth of the iliac crest. This type of injury is rare and generally occurs in an older child or young adolescent since the average age of closure of the apophysis is 16 years. An avulsion or fracture of the iliac apophysis may result from a sudden severe contraction of the abdominal muscles during a twisting injury or with abrupt directional changes while running. Radiographs are recommended for the immature athlete who has pain in the region of the iliac crest following a twisting injury.

The second condition to be considered in the differential diagnosis of a hip pointer is a strain of the external oblique aponeurosis. This injury involves tearing of the insertion of the abdominal musculature onto the iliac crest. The injury is often caused by forceful contraction of the abdominal muscles while the trunk of the body is being forced to the contralateral side. The diagnosis can be made when the player has both localized lateral abdominal tenderness and pain with trunk flexion to the opposite side. Contracture of the lateral abdominal muscles against resistance should also cause pain. Differentiation from a hip pointer should not be difficult, as functional movement of the muscles attached to the iliac crest does not significantly increase pain in a hip pointer.

## TREATMENT

Treatment of a hip pointer on the day of injury is aimed at minimizing the amount of slow bleeding into the surrounding tissues. Recommended treatment includes rest and the intermittent application of ice for 20- to 30-minute periods with a 4-inch or 6-inch elastic wrap over the first 24 to 48 hours, depending on the severity of the symptoms. The use of heat, massage, or vigorous physical therapy should be delayed during this period because of the possibility of increasing the bleeding. The use of crutches with partial weight bearing of the involved extremity may be beneficial for several days in cases of severe limping. Referral to a physician is necessary in cases of persistent symptoms of severe pain that are unresponsive to the above measures over a short period of time. Clancy states that soluble steroid injection into the area of injury within the first several hours has demonstrated marked alleviation of symptoms that normally are incapacitating for 5 to 7 days. Injection performed a day after injury appears to have no benefit.

## REHABILITATION AND RETURN-TO-PLAY CRITERIA

Rehabilitation is aimed at regaining hip and trunk motion through gentle stretching exercises after the initial discomfort has subsided. Ice massage and ultrasound may be beneficial during this period after stretching. Once motion has been regained, light jogging can be started. The player is gradually allowed to resume all noncontact activities as tolerated, with the application of ice to the injured area recommended after practice. Recovery time will vary from several days to several weeks depending on the extent of the injury. Return to contact activities is allowed when there are no significant symptoms referable to the area of injury, even after a vigorous noncontact workout. As the athlete returns to contact in practice and game situations, a protective pad will be required in addition to properly fitted routine pads. Prevention of these disabling contusions to the pelvis, by periodically checking that the athlete has properly positioned pads during play, is most important.

## GROIN STRAIN

The groin strain involves injury to the adductor musculature as it originates from the pelvis. This injury is common in sports requiring quick changes in direction (football and soccer) and in sports in which the adductors are required for propulsion (skating and hockey).

### MECHANISM OF INJURY

In football the groin strain occurs most commonly as a result of forced external rotation of the abducted leg. This mechanism can occur through tackling or from a player slipping on a muddy field. A less common mechanism of injury can involve forced abduction of the thigh, as in a straddling injury.

### CLINICAL DIAGNOSIS

The athlete with an adductor strain will have localized point tenderness evident along the subcutaneous edge of the pubic ramus. Occasionally a palpable defect in the adductor origin may be present. Passive abduction of the thigh will elicit pain. The "adductor test" can be performed, in which the athlete lays on his or her back and attempts to forcibly adduct the legs against the trainer's resistance, eliciting groin pain.

## TREATMENT

Initial treatment of a groin strain includes rest with the application of ice and use of antiinflammatory agents. A 6-inch elastic wrap is commonly used to provide compression. The athlete's hip may be strapped in a spica wrap with the thigh flexed and slightly externally rotated. Following the acute period of injury, treatment modalities—such as warm whirlpool or ultrasound, as well as gentle stretching exercises—are beneficial. Active range of motion exercises are performed with the athlete lying on the side of the body and are started early to maintain a normal range of motion. Resistive exercises, including adductor isometrics (as in squeezing a medicine ball), can be started 3 weeks after the injury. The goal of rehabilitation of a groin strain is slow, gradual stretching and strengthening of the injured area. If significant pain is still present after 1 week on attempted running, and there is no evidence of fracture or complete rupture, Clancy recommends injection of 1 ml of dexamethasone (Decadron) (4 mg/ml) into the affected area.

## RETURN-TO-PLAY CRITERIA

The athlete should avoid running, jumping, or climbing stairs while symptomatic following a groin strain. Recovery time will vary depending on the extent of the injury. Once the athlete is able to perform stretching and strengthening exercises without pain, the running program may be started. The athlete may return to play when he or she is able to demonstrate the ability to run and cut according to the running program (see the Appendix on p. 255) and when there is a normal range of motion and flexibility of the involved hip. The athlete can be taught a program of home exercises for adductor stretching and strengthening to prevent recurrence.

## AVULSION FRACTURES ABOUT THE PELVIS

Within any given musculotendinous unit, injury may occur as a strain within the body of the muscle, at the muscle-tendon junction, at the tendon's insertion into bone, or by avulsion of the bone containing the insertion of the tendon. In adults the most common location of strain is at the muscle-tendon junction, whereas in adolescents bony avulsion of the tendon insertion is more common. All avulsion fractures share a similar mechanism of injury that involves sudden severe contraction of the associated muscle, which detaches from the pelvis with a fragment of bone. These injuries occur most commonly between the ages of 14 and 17 and are more common among boys than among girls.

The following regions are the most common sites of avulsion:

- The ischial tuberosity by the attachment of the hamstring muscles
- The anterosuperior iliac spine by the attachment of the sartorius muscle
- The anteroinferior iliac spine by the attachment of the rectus femoris muscle
- The iliac apophysis by the abdominal muscle attachments (discussed in the section on hip pointers)
- The lesser trochanter of the femur by the attachment of the iliopsoas muscle

## CLINICAL DIAGNOSIS

Severe pain is experienced by the athlete at the site of bony avulsion. Localized tenderness and swelling are often present. Pain is accentuated by resisted action of the involved musculotendinous unit.

## TREATMENT

Treatment on the field consists of the application of ice to the affected area, along with compression.

A five-stage progression for treatment of avulsion fractures has been described:

| | |
|---|---|
| Phase I | Rest with positioning to relax the involved muscles; ice application; analgesic medication. |
| Phase II | When acute pain has subsided, gradually increase excursion of the injured musculotendinous unit with gentle stretching exercises. |
| Phase III | When full active range of motion is achieved, begin a comprehensive progressive resistance program. |
| Phase IV | When 50% of strength returns, integrate the use of the injured musculotendinous unit with the other muscles of the pelvis and lower extremity by conditioning exercises for all muscle groups. The athlete starts with stationary bicycling and walking and progresses to jogging during this phase. |
| Phase V | The athlete may return to competitive sports when there is full hip range of motion and full strength by isokinetic testing, and when the athlete demonstrates agility in running and cutting. |

Clinical healing of an avulsion fracture usually occurs after 3 to 6 weeks. The recovery time necessary before allowing an athlete to return to play varies from 4 to 8 weeks. Avulsion fractures of the anterior or inferior iliac spines rarely require surgery. Avulsions of the ischial tuberosity may require surgical fixation.

## SNAPPING HIP

The onset of the "snapping" hip is usually insidious, without any known antecedent injury. The snapping sensation results from the iliotibial band snapping over the greater trochanter of the femur.

### MECHANISM OF INJURY
Repetitive motion causes inflammation of the iliotibial band as it passes over the greater trochanter. Inflammation leads to thickening and fibrosis of the iliotibial band and increases the snapping sensation.

### CLINICAL DIAGNOSIS
The athlete will report a "snapping" sensation in the involved hip. Local tenderness to palpation of the greater trochanteric region may be present. The diagnosis is confirmed if the athlete can reproduce the snapping with weight bearing while the examiner's hand is held over the lateral aspect of the hip near the greater trochanter.

### TREATMENT
On-field treatment recommendations include resting the athlete and applying ice and compression to the area of tenderness.

Rehabilitation includes ultrasound or ice therapy to the area of maximum tenderness. A program of iliotibial band stretching exercises is started after acute symptoms of pain have subsided. Progression to generalized conditioning and lower extremity strengthening exercises occurs before the athlete returns to activities that include running.

### RETURN-TO-PLAY CRITERIA
The athlete is allowed to return to play when full strength and range of motion of the hip are present and when the athlete is able to perform the running and cutting exercises outlined in the running program. (See the Appendix on p. 255.)

### Bibliography
Merrifield HH, Cowan RF: Groin strain injuries in ice hockey, *Am J Sports Med* 1:41-42, 1973.
Metzmaker JN, Pappas AM: Avulsion fractures of the pelvis, *Am J Sports Med* 13:349-358, 1985.

Sim FH, Scott CG: Injuries of the pelvis and hip in athletes: anatomy and function. In Nicholas JA, Hershman EB: *The lower extremity and spine in sports medicine,* St Louis, 1986, Mosby–Year Book.

Waters P, Mills M: Hip and pelvic injuries in the young athlete, *Clin Sports Med* 7:513-526, 1988.

Wootton JR, Cross NJ, Holt KW: Avulsion of the ischial apophysis: the case for open reduction and internal fixation, *J Bone Joint Surg* 72B:625-627, 1990.

# Chapter 12

# Injuries to the thigh

Michael A. Sclafani

Proper on-field evaluation of thigh injuries requires a basic under-standing of regional anatomy and a knowledge of the most common types of injuries. The upper leg contains a single bone—the femur—and three major muscle groups: the quadriceps, the hamstrings, and the adductors. Both the quadriceps and the hamstrings are two-joint muscles that attach on the pelvis and the tibia. Injuries to these muscles can therefore cause restriction of both hip and knee motion. This chapter focuses on contu-sions and strains of the quadriceps and hamstring muscles, and fractures of the femur. Adductor muscle strains are covered in Chapter 11.

## QUADRICEPS CONTUSION

A contusion of the quadriceps muscle is one of the most common sports injuries of the thigh. The spectrum of injury can range from a very mild contusion, after which the athlete continues to compete, to a severely damaged muscle with a resultant complication of myositis ossificans.

### MECHANISM OF INJURY

A quadriceps contusion results from a direct external blow to the ante-rior, medial, or lateral aspect of the thigh. The severity of the injury is proportional to the amount of compressive force, the total area over which the force is applied, and the resistance of the thigh tissues.[9]

### CLINICAL DIAGNOSIS

The athlete complains of a dull, aching pain in the thigh that is aggra-vated by hip or knee flexion. Depending on the severity of injury, some players continue to compete, only complaining of symptoms after the game is completed. Most individuals have more severe pain, swelling, and stiffness the day after the injury occurs.

Physical examination of the thigh reveals diffuse tenderness in the region of the blow. The muscle may be in spasm, and passive flexion of the hip or knee exacerbates the pain. Ecchymosis may be present.

Classification of injury is based on the limitation of knee flexion and alteration in gait as follows[4]:

| | |
|---|---|
| Grade I (mild) | Knee flexion greater than 90 degrees |
| | No alteration in gait |
| Grade II (moderate) | Knee flexion between 45 and 90 degrees |
| | Antalgic gait |
| Grade III (severe) | Knee flexion less than 45 degrees |
| | Severe limp |

## DIFFERENTIAL DIAGNOSIS

**Quadriceps muscle-tendon rupture**

The patient is unable to actively extend the knee, and a palpable defect can be felt.

**Femoral stress fracture**

The patient has more localized, point tenderness, usually in the subtrochanteric region.

## TREATMENT

Initial treatment should focus on minimizing hemorrhage, swelling, and spasm. The hip and knee should be kept flexed to tolerance to prevent subsequent extension contracture.[8] The thigh should be wrapped with a 6-inch Ace wrap. Ice packs should be placed over the injured area and held in place with another elastic bandage. A patient with a grade III contusion should be given crutches and allowed to bear weight as tolerated.

An athlete should be referred to a local sports medicine clinic if a grade III injury is diagnosed or if swelling and pain worsen over the next few days. A sympathetic knee effusion is usually apparent a few days after a significant grade II or grade III injury.

After the initial phase of hemorrhage control is completed, treatment should focus on restoration of pain-free motion, strength, and endurance.

## RETURN-TO-PLAY CRITERIA

The athlete can return to competition only after he or she regains full functional range of motion and adequate muscle strength, and is able to complete the running program. (See the Appendix on p. 255.) There should be no pain in response to palpation of the affected area. The athlete should be rechecked for loss of motion several days after beginning the running program. If some loss of flexion is noted, the athlete should be placed back on his or her rehabilitation program.

If an athlete with a grade III quadriceps contusion develops myositis ossificans, he or she cannot return to play until the area shows complete inculcation of the myositis ossificans with sclerotic shell, and until the area is totally nontender to palpation and there is full range of motion.

The average disability time has been shown to be 13 days for mild, 19 days for moderate, and 21 days for severe contusions.[8]

On return to contact sports, a large thigh pad is recommended to prevent reinjury.

## HAMSTRING STRAIN

A muscle strain results from an overstretching or excessively tensile force that causes damage at the musculotendinous junction. The hamstring muscles—semitendinosus, semimembranosus, and biceps femoris—are the most susceptible muscles in the thigh to strain injuries.

### MECHANISM OF INJURY

The major cause of hamstring strains is a sudden, forced change in the length of the musculotendinous unit. This often occurs during sprinting, when flexion of the hip and extension of the knee place the muscle under maximal stretch.[6] The hamstring muscles also function to decelerate leg swing, and they may be injured when an athlete suddenly changes direction or starts to slow down. Risk factors for hamstring strains include lack of flexibility, an abnormal quadriceps/hamstring ratio, and poor form.[6] The short head of the biceps femoris is the most commonly strained hamstring muscle.

### CLINICAL DIAGNOSIS

Depending on the severity of injury, the patient may continue to compete or may immediately grab the back of the leg, fall to the ground, and need help off the field.

Classification of the spectrum of muscle strain injuries has been made by O'Donoghue.[7] In a first degree (or mild) strain, there is no significant loss of strength or motion. The patient usually continues to compete and only complains of muscle soreness after he or she cools down.

A second degree (or moderate) strain is a partial tear of muscle fibers resulting in any degree of incomplete strength loss. The athlete often claims to have felt or heard a "pop." With the patient prone and the knee partially flexed, palpation can locate the site of injury. Ecchymosis may also be evident.

A third degree (or severe) strain is a complete rupture of the musculotendinous unit that results in major hemorrhage and complete loss of function.

## ON-FIELD TREATMENT

Initial treatment should focus on minimizing hemorrhage and spasm. Ice has been shown to cause vasoconstriction, decrease bleeding, and produce anesthesia of the area.[5] The thigh is wrapped with a 6-inch Ace wrap, and ice packs are held in place with another elastic bandage. Compressive wraps should not be too tight, to prevent distal edema formation. Protection of the injured muscle by using crutches is recommended for moderate to severe injuries. If by 7 to 10 days postinjury there is still appreciable pain and loss of function, an injection of 1 ml of soluble corticosteroid (dexamethasone [Decadron] 4 mg/ml) is considered.

## RETURN-TO-PLAY CRITERIA

After the first 24 to 48 hours, depending on the degree of strain, treatment should progress to gentle stretching and isometric exercises. All rehabilitation exercises should be performed in the pain-free range of motion. When the athlete is free of pain and has a complete range of motion of the hip and knee, the running program is instituted. (See the Appendix on p. 255.) After completing the running program, the patient is allowed to return to competition. Most athletes with mild sprains can return to play in 2 to 3 days. Athletes with severe strains are often sidelined for 2 to 3 weeks, if correct therapeutic measures are followed.

## MYOSITIS OSSIFICANS

Myositis ossificans is abnormal bone formation or calcium deposits that develop in a previously injured muscle. The heterotopic ossification may or may not be attached to the underlying bone.

## MECHANISM OF INJURY

Myositis ossificans usually develops 2 to 4 weeks after a single severe blow, or multiple blows, to the quadriceps muscle. A few cases of ectopic bone formation after a quadriceps strain have been reported.[3]

## CLINICAL DIAGNOSIS

The athlete complains of pain and swelling in a localized area of his or her thigh and is usually able to recall a previous traumatic episode. On examination, a palpable tender mass may be felt. The athlete may also lack some knee flexion.

## ON-FIELD TREATMENT

As with thigh contusions, the athlete should be treated with rest, ice, and elevation. All athletes with suspected myositis ossificans should be referred to a local sports medicine facility. Radiographs and careful follow-up are essential to rule out a possible malignancy.

## RETURN-TO-PLAY CRITERIA

When the athlete has full, painless range of motion of the hip and knee—and when the injured area is no longer painful in response to palpation—the running program is started. (See the Appendix on p. 255.) After completion of the running program, the patient is allowed to return to competition. On return to contact sports, the athlete must use a protective thigh pad to prevent reinjury.

# FEMORAL STRESS FRACTURE

Stress fractures of the femur are an uncommon cause of thigh pain in the athlete. As compared with acute fractures of the femur—which are due to violent, high-energy trauma and cause immediate pain and obvious deformity—stress fractures can mimic other painful conditions of the thigh.

## MECHANISM OF INJURY

Stress fractures result from repetitive overloading of bone that results in a microscopic disruption of cortical continuity.[2] These fractures usually occur in the athlete who is participating in lengthy training sessions or who suddenly increases his or her training intensity. The most common sites of involvement are the proximal and distal aspects of the femur, such as the femoral neck, subtrochanteric, and supracondylar regions.

## CLINICAL DIAGNOSIS

Most athletes with stress fractures complain of a low-grade aching in the thigh. Palpation causes local tenderness at the fracture site. There is usually only mild swelling, no limited range of motion, and no obvious deformity. While pain may be present only during athletic activity, it eventually progresses to affect normal gait. If left untreated or if the athlete does not get medical care, the fracture can displace, resulting in more severe pain and deformity.[1]

## ON-FIELD TREATMENT

Athletes with suspected femoral stress fractures should be placed, non–weight bearing, on crutches and referred to a regional medical center. Plain radiographs are usually normal the first 3 to 6 weeks after the onset of pain, and diagnosis depends on a positive radioisotope bone scan.

## RETURN-TO-PLAY CRITERIA

Athletes are placed on crutches and allowed toe-touch weight bearing for the first 4 weeks of treatment. The crutches are discontinued when the athlete is able to ambulate pain-free. Lower body strengthening is initiated and progresses to low-impact activities such as biking and swimming. If radiographs show evidence of callus formation—and the athlete remains pain free—the running program is initiated at 6 to 8 weeks after the injury. The athlete is allowed to return to competition after pain-free completion of the running program. (See the Appendix on p. 255.)

### References

1. Bargren JH, Tilson DH, Bridgeford OE: Prevention of displaced fatigue fractures of the femur, *J Bone Joint Surg* 53A:1115-1117, 1971.
2. Butler JE, Braun SL, McConnell BG: Subtrochanteric stress fractures in runners, *Am J Sports Med* 10:228-232, 1982.
3. Jackson DW: Managing myositis ossificans, *Physician Sports Med*, pp 56-61, 1975.
4. Jackson DW, Feagin JA: Quadriceps contusions in young athletes, *J Bone Joint Surg* 55A:95-105, 1973.
5. McMaster WC: A literary review of ice therapy in injuries, *Am J Sports Med* 5:124-126, 1977.
6. Nicholas JA, Hershman EB: *The lower extremity and spine in sports medicine*, St Louis, 1986, Mosby–Year Book.
7. O'Donoghue DH: *Treatment of injuries to athletes*, ed 4, Philadelphia, 1984, WB Saunders.
8. Ryan JB, Wheeler JH et al: Quadriceps contusions: West Point update, *Am J Sports Med* 19:299-304, 1991.
9. Zarins B, Ciullo JV: Acute muscle and tendon injuries in athletes, *Clin Sports Med* 2:167-182, 1983.

# Chapter 13

# Knee injuries

Scott David Martin
William G. Clancy, Jr.

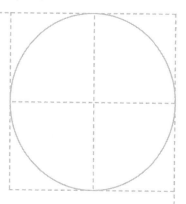

## EVALUATION OF THE ACUTELY INJURED KNEE

### HISTORY

The proper on-field evaluation of any athletic injury begins with the awareness of how the injury occurred. By astute observation of the mechanism of injury, one can be cognizant of a potentially severe injury that might otherwise be dismissed as trivial at first glance. After determining the mechanism of injury, an open mind should be kept so as not to miss an associated injury or misinterpret a physical finding by focusing on a particular diagnosis. If direct observation of the injury did not occur, the athlete should be questioned about the mechanism of injury. Current symptoms including the severity of pain, extent of disability, feeling of instability, and any prior injury to the affected knee should be noted. The athlete should be questioned about the specific incident surrounding the injury, such as the position of the leg, any feeling of "giving out" or instability, or the presence of an audible "pop" or "click" with an associated sharp pain.

### PHYSICAL EXAMINATION

Most knee injuries can be divided into overuse injuries or noncontact and acute traumatic injuries. Overuse injuries usually occur insidiously over time, as a result of a repetitive number of relatively small loads. They are characterized by pain, tenderness, and other inflammatory conditions.[13] Traumatic injuries occur acutely as a result of a massive overload to the knee. This chapter concentrates on the acutely injured knee; however, one must keep in mind that an acute exacerbation of an overuse injury can also occur.

The initial evaluation of an acutely injured athlete should take place on the playing field to ascertain the severity of the injury. A complete examination must be performed so as not to overlook any injuries. Both knees should always be examined for comparison. Following examination of the normal knee with the determination of the overall laxity and range of motion, attention is directed to the injured knee. Physical examination should begin with observation and the position of the limb. Assessment of the injured limb should compare it with the contralateral limb for any subtle differences. Any gross abnormalities should be noted, such as swelling, deformity, obvious bleeding, or ecchymosis. The neurovascular status of the injured extremity should be assessed, especially if there is any deformity or significant swelling.

Knee stability is tested toward the end of the exam, so as not to cause guarding with quadriceps and hamstring spasm and decreased patient cooperation (which can mask an unstable knee). The uninjured knee is examined first to determine the overall physiologic joint laxity. The sequence (from least stressful to most stressful) of tests that is preferred by the senior author (Clancy) is as follows: Lachman's test; the anterior and posterior drawer tests; the varus-valgus test at 30 and 0 degrees; the pivot shift test; and the reverse pivot shift test.

## TRAUMATIC INJURIES OF THE KNEE

### MEDIAL COLLATERAL LIGAMENT INJURY
#### Pathophysiology
An isolated medial collateral ligament (MCL) injury usually occurs when a valgus (outside) force is applied to the knee with the foot planted (Fig. 13-1). This frequently occurs during a clipping injury to the knee. The resulting force causes gapping of the medial joint line with stretching and tearing of the MCL fibers. This injury can also occur as part of a complex ligamentous injury with concomitant involvement of the anterior and/or posterior cruciate ligaments, in addition to a meniscal tear.

#### On-field evaluation
On physical examination, there is usually localized swelling and tenderness to palpation over the site of injury to the ligament on the medial (inside) of the knee. There may be a palpable defect at the site of the torn ligament, with visible ecchymosis from the resulting subcutaneous hemorrhage. Oftentimes the athlete will find it difficult to completely extend the knee secondary to pain—opting instead to keep the knee slightly flexed, which relaxes the MCL. This lack of extension secondary to pain should be differentiated from a mechanical block caused by a displaced bucket handle tear of the meniscus. There is often increased pain with valgus stressing to the knee.

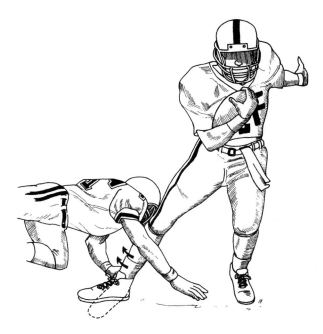

**Fig. 13-1.** Valgus external rotational force produced by a blow to the outside of the knee with the foot planted.

An MCL injury can be graded according to the amount of medial joint space opening that is present when a valgus (or outside) stress is applied to the knee at 30 degrees of flexion and with the knee in extension with neutral rotation. Examination should always begin with the uninjured knee to determine the natural laxity of the knee.

**Grade I injury.** There is 0 to 5 mm of opening with the knee flexed at 30 degrees. There may be some attenuation of fibers without plastic deformation and no loss of continuity. Therefore the amount of increased knee laxity as compared with the opposite knee is insignificant.

**Grade II injury.** There is 5 to 10 mm of opening, with partial disruption of ligament fibers.

**Grade III injury.** There is greater than 10 mm of opening, with complete disruption of all fibers and with instability and laxity present but no opening in extension.

The senior author finds this classification system to be incomplete and has added an additional grade to accurately describe the possible extent of this injury.

**Grade IV injury.** There is significant instability and laxity at 30 degrees and mild to moderate laxity in neutral extension to valgus stressing, which indicates complete disruption of the MCL and a complete tear of the posterior oblique ligament. When this amount of laxity is present at 0 degrees of extension, there is usually (but not always) an associated injury to the anterior cruciate ligament (ACL), the posterior cruciate ligament (PCL), or both.

**Treatment**

Acutely, the knee is usually splinted in full extension, which provides the greatest amount of knee stability. The knee should be wrapped with a compressive dressing and iced; weight bearing should be protected with crutches. The athlete should be referred to a qualified physician or sports medicine facility.

O'Donoghue popularized early surgical repair of grade III sprains, followed by a postoperative period of rigid immobilization.[51] Since then, success in nonoperative treatment with earlier mobilization has led to an aggressive rehabilitation approach to even isolated grade III MCL sprains.[19,50]

The senior author's approach to isolated grade I and II MCL sprains involves early compression and icing until pain and swelling have subsided (usually 48 to 72 hours). Grade I and II sprains are then treated without immobilization, and athletes with these types of injuries are started on early mobilization with progressive strengthening exercises. Grade III strains are treated with a knee immobilizer for the first week, after which intermittent immobilization is carried out until painless motion is present between 5 and 100 degrees and the patient is able to ambulate with minimal or no limp. The athlete is started on quadriceps sets and leg lifts on the second day postinjury. When the patient has 90 degrees of painless flexion, a progressive weight training program is initiated. Water exercises are begun on the third or fourth day whenever possible. When the athlete has full painless range of motion, he or she is started on a functional running program that must be completed in its entirety and comfortably before the athlete is allowed to return to competition. (See the Appendix on p. 255.)

When there is a complete tear of the ACL (as evidenced by a positive Lachman's test) or a complete tear of the PCL (as evidenced by a complete loss of the tibial plateau step-off at 90 degrees of knee flexion), along with a complete disruption of the MCL, a complex ligamentous injury exists. In this case, there is usually significant valgus laxity at 0 degrees of extension, and it can be assumed there has been a complete tear of both the tibial collateral ligament (the anterior half of the MCL) and the posterior oblique ligament (the posterior half of the MCL). When this occurs, there has been enough joint distraction to allow the tibial collateral ligament to flip anterior to the pes anserine tendons—preventing proper healing if not treated surgically. The senior author refers to this condition as the "Stener lesion" of the knee. Similarly, the posterior oblique fibers may roll up superiorly (like a window shade) to the level of the medial epicondyle. For these two reasons, complete tears of both portions of the MCL (anterior and posterior obliques) need to be surgically treated when associated with a complete tear of either cruciate ligament.

## ANTERIOR CRUCIATE LIGAMENT INJURY
### Pathophysiology
The ACL primarily prevents anterior subluxation or displacement of the tibia on the femur. The typical mechanism of injury for a tear of the ACL occurs with activities involving deceleration, jumping, or cutting actions. In jumping activities, the injury usually results from a mislanding that causes the knee to go out. In football a valgus, or outside, rotational force to a planted knee (such as occurs during clipping) may result in an ACL tear. Another example of this type of force that produces an ACL tear is seen in downhill skiiing with a twisting fall. Frequently, there may be involvment of more than one ligamentous structure of the knee, in addition to a meniscal tear.

### On-field evaluation
Acute ACL disruptions are usually associated with a tense hemarthrosis. Frequently, the swelling may take 24 hours to become evident.[59] The ACL is partially or completely torn more than 70% of the time when associated with a traumatic hemarthrosis.[59] Approximately 40% of the time there is an associated "pop" at the time of injury.[62] Oftentimes the knee will abruptly give out, causing the athelte to fall to the ground or floor.

On palpation of the knee there is frequently pain along the anterolateral and anteromedial joint line. The MCL is often torn at the same time; palpation may reveal tenderness anywhere from the proximal to distal attachements, signifying disruption. Lachman's test is very accurate in determining the integrity of the ACL. The test is performed with the athlete supine and the examiner on the same side as the affected knee. The knee is flexed 20 degrees, and the upper hand is grasped around the outside of the distal thigh while the lower hand is grasped around the inside of the proximal tibial region. The tibia is then translated anteriorly with the lower hand while stabilizing the femur with the upper hand. As with any part of the physical exam, the overall laxity should be compared with the contralateral knee. One of the most common reasons for a false negative Lachman's test is hamstring spasm and/or a displaced bucket handle tear of the medial meniscus.

### Treatment
For an athlete who has experienced a twisting injury with a concomitant hemarthrosis, an ACL injury should be suspected until proven otherwise.

Initial treatment involves applying ice and a compressive dressing, and splinting the leg in a comfortable position. The athlete should be kept on protective weight bearing with crutches until evaluated by a physician. Any athlete that is complaining of recurrent instability or giving way with twisting, pivoting, running, or deceleration should be suspected of having a major knee ligament injury and should be referred to a physician with training in sports medicine injuries. Without the appropriate treatment, recurrent instability may occur, with resulting damage to the internal structures of the knee.[21]

The natural history of an ACL-deficient knee usually leads to progessive anatomic and functional deterioration.* In addition, meniscal degeneration and secondary stretching of ligamentous restraints may lead to eventual osteoarthritis.[20,33,41,42,54] There are relatively few studies in the literature comparing the outcome of patients who have ACL reconstruction with those patients treated nonoperatively.† Still, most authors would agree there is a high-risk patient who should be treated with early reconstruction and a low-risk patient who may be managed conservatively.[15,48,59,61] The athlete with an ACL-deficient knee is at risk for functional impairment, secondary meniscal tear, and development of joint arthrosis.

The goal of ACL reconstruction is to restore normal joint stability, and to return the patient to full function and prevent secondary joint injury and arthrosis. Some authors believe certain patients can be treated conservatively without sustaining secondary joint injury.‡ ACL reconstruction in properly selected patients will significantly decrease the likelihood of recurrent knee instability and further knee injury.

Athletes with ACL-deficient knees that are treated conservatively after injury are started on a rehabilitation program. In the first few weeks of the program isometric hamstring and quadriceps exercises are initiated until pain and swelling have subsided. The second phase of the program begins after 3 weeks, and the athlete is progressed to isokinetic exercises and cycling. The final phase of the program usually starts about 4 to 6 weeks after the initial injury and concentrates on endurance and strengthening exercises. Once there is significant gain in functional activity and confidence the athlete is gradually progessed to competition.

## POSTERIOR CRUCIATE LIGAMENT INJURY
### Pathophysiology
The PCL is probably more frequently injured than realized. A direct blow to the flexed knee is usually the most common mechanism of

---

*References 8, 21, 39, 42, 45, 46, 49.
†References 2, 3, 23, 25, 29, 31, 43.
‡References 23, 25, 31, 32, 49, 53, 58.

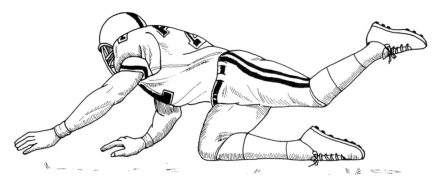

**Fig. 13-2.** Posteriorly directed force to the proximal tibia that is produced by a fall on the flexed knee with the foot in plantar flexion.

injury.[52] This injury is best exemplified when an athlete falls to the ground or floor on a flexed knee with a plantarflexed foot (Fig. 13-2). A second mechanism of injury is a fall with hyperflexion of the knee. This mechanism, in our experience, not infrequently produces an interstitial or in situ failure. The PCL injury can also occur from a hyperextension of the knee; when this occurs, it is usually associated with ACL disruption and/or knee dislocation.[36,52] This can result from a direct blow to the front of the tibia in an extended knee or as a misstep while running or jumping.

**On-field evaluation**

Injuries of the PCL are often subtle and are frequently missed in an acute setting. In Clancy and colleagues' series of PCL injury studies, approximately one half of the injuries were isolated and the other one half were complex.[9] Usually there is only a mild effusion with little discomfort. There is often increasing pain with knee flexion past 90 degrees.

In evaluating the knee, first examine the normal or contralateral knee by palpating the step-off. This is done by flexing the knee to 90 degrees (with the tibia in neutral rotation) and palpating the anteromedial and anterolateral tibial plateau step-off, which is usually about 10 mm. Then examine the injured knee. If the step-off is less than the normal knee but is still palpable, it can be considered a +1 posterior subluxation or translation and indicates PCL laxity. If the anterior tibial plateau is flush with medial and lateral femoral condyles, then there is a +2 posterior subluxation. If the anterior tibial plateau is posterior to the femoral condyles, then there is a +3 posterior subluxation that indicates complete disruption of the PCL. With the knee kept at 80 to 90 degrees of flexion and the foot in neutral rotation, a posterior drawer test is performed. Both hands are grasped around the proximal tibia, just below the joint line, and the tibia is pushed posteriorly. Increased translation posteriorly, when compared with the contralateral knee, signifies a PCL injury.[26, 27]

**Treatment**

The PCL is the strongest and most important ligament of the knee, providing 95% of the total restraint to posterior displacement of the tibia. However, there is no consensus about its treatment, as a review of the literature will quickly suggest.* On-field treatment is similar to that for other knee ligamentous injuries. Initial treatment involves applying ice and a compressive dressing, and splinting the leg in full extension. The athlete should be kept on protective weight bearing with crutches until evaluated by a physician.

We currently treat all complex ligamentous injuries involving the PCL. In isolated cases the treatment is tailored to the individual patient, with operative indications based on the degeree of laxity and symptoms, and on the patient's age, activity level, and overall demands. Our investigations, as well as those of others, suggest that the nonoperative approach to isolated PCL tears may lead to increasing degenerative changes in the knee over time, in addition to progressive subjective complaints.[9,12,35] Other studies report satisfactory short- and long-term functional results with nonoperative treatment.[22,52,56]

A nonoperative PCL rehabilitation program begins with quadriceps sets, straight leg raises, and mini squats from 0 to 45 degrees. After a few weeks the athlete is progressed to cycling (to improve range of motion), and a pool program is started. By 4 to 5 weeks after the initial injury, the athlete is progressed to a Stairmaster, knee extension exercises from 90 to 30 degrees, and light resistance hamstring curls. In the final phase of the program, which is usually around the sixth or seventh week after injury, running is initiated. The athlete is gradually returned to sports activity if there is no pain, tenderness, or swelling on clinical exam and no recurrent instability with increased functional demands.

## MENISCAL INJURY

### Pathophysiology

Meniscal injuries may result from a rather insignificant movement such as twisting or squatting, or they may be associated with a more serious ligamentous injury that occurs with more severe trauma to the knee.[14] Tears of the medial meniscus are more common than lateral tears because of the semicircular shape of the meniscus and medial plateau and decreased mobility of the medial meniscus (Fig. 13-3). In individuals less than 30 years old, a longitudinal or bucket handle tear is more common; whereas in individuals over 40, horizontal (or flap) tears are seen more frequently.

---

*References 9, 12, 25, 35, 52, 56.

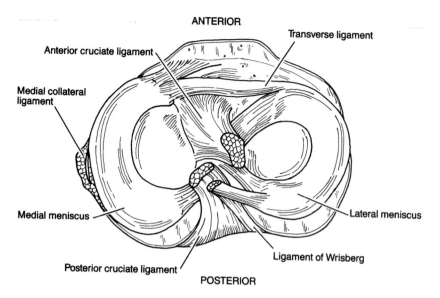

**Fig. 13-3.** A cross-sectional anatomic view of the knee.

## On-field evaluation

In isolated cases of meniscal injuries, the symptoms may seem insignificant, with very little pain or swelling. Oftentimes, there is a delayed onset of swelling, which results from a synovial reaction to the meniscal injury. Locking of the knee may occur with a bucket handle tear and is caused by a mechanical block to flexion or extension of the knee by the torn meniscus. If the torn portion of the meniscus becomes completely displaced, there may be no loss of motion and very little pain.

## Treatment

If there is an apparent mechanical block to the athlete's extension, the knee should be splinted and weight bearing should be protected with crutches until the athlete is evaluated by a physician. If the athlete returns to play but continues to complain of locking, catching, or giving way of the knee, a meniscal injury should be considered and the athlete should be referred to a sports medicine center.

In 1948, Fairbanks reported on the disappointing late consequences of total meniscectomy.[57] Since then, clinical and basic science research has defined the critical role of the menisci in the complex biomechanics of the knee and has underscored the importance of preserving these structures whenever possible.*

---

*References 1, 4, 7, 10, 11, 24, 34, 37, 38, 47, 55.

Treatment of meniscal tears has been greatly aided by arthroscopy. Currently, the basic clinical principle is to preserve as much functioning meniscal tissue while addressing the clinical symptoms caused by the meniscal tear.[19] Over the past decade, meniscal repair has evolved as a method to salvage a torn meniscus whenever possible.*

## PATELLAR SUBLUXATION OR DISLOCATION
### Pathophysiology

A subluxation of the patella, or knee cap, occurs when the patella does not ride within the trochlear groove of the femur but is displaced partially out of the groove. A dislocation of the patella occurs when the patella is completely displaced out of the trochlear groove.

Patellar dislocations are rarely caused by contact injuries, but rather they occur as the result of external rotation of the leg, active contraction of the quadriceps, and knee extension. The athlete may have a propensity for patellar subluxation or dislocation because of biomechanical variation, including femoral anteversion, external tibial torsion, genu valgum (knock knee), and hyperpronation of the feet. The injury usually occurs during weight bearing; however, there have been reported cases of patellar dislocation in the unloaded knee during gymnastics and diving.

### On-field evaluation

Frequently the athlete hears a tearing or ripping type of noise. The injury is usually associated with significant swelling caused by a large hemarthrosis. There is frequently ecchymosis located over the medial side of the knee caused by tearing of the vastus medialis from the medial intermuscular septum. In addition, there is usually significant pain to palpation of the intermuscular septum just above the adductor tubercle.

There is often significant pain and quadriceps spasm with any attempted range of motion, and the athlete has difficulty bearing weight on the affected extremity. Tenderness can be elicited by palpating the medial side of the knee over the region of the medial intermuscular septum. Pain may also be elicited by palpating the medial facet of the patella, which is frequently injured during traumatic dislocation. Because of the significant pain, swelling, and quadriceps spasm, it is difficult to assess ligamentous integrity acutely.

### Treatment

If the dislocated patella does not spontaneously relocate, the knee will appear grossly deformed, with the patella off to the lateral or outside of the knee. If this occurs, the patella may be relocated by slowly extending the knee while putting pressure on the outside of the patella. If relocation does not occur, the knee should be splinted in a comfortable position

---

*References 5-7, 16-18, 28, 30, 40, 44.

and the athlete transported to an emergency room or sports medicine facility.

If the patella is relocated, the knee is immobilized in the position of comfort. Ice, local compression, and protected weight bearing with crutches should be instituted. Aspiration is rarely indicated since it is the senior author's experience that the hemarthrosis is likely to occur after aspiration. The patient should be referred to a qualified physician or sports medicine facility. Radiographs are frequently indicated to rule out an intraarticular fracture or fracture of the medial facet of the patella, which is not uncommon with traumatic dislocation.

Definitive treatment is aimed at reestablishing quadriceps strength while protecting the knee against subsequent dislocations. Isometric quadriceps exercises are initiated as soon as possible. An electrical muscle-stimulating unit may be helpful in maintaining quadriceps bulk early on. Active range of motion exercises are initiated at 1 week postinjury. A knee immobilizer is used until swelling has subsided and the athlete has painless flexion of 100 degrees with normal gait. At this point the patient is weaned from a knee immobilizer, which is then replaced with a neoprene sleeve with a lateral pad. The sleeve is used until the athlete has a normal gait, after which it is worn during athletic activity for at least 6 months or until the athlete feels confident playing without the brace.

Sometimes patellar dislocation, and more commonly patellar subluxation, may become a chronic problem. If this occurs, the patient is started on a vigorous physical therapy program. If the patient continues to have problems surgery may be needed.

## REHABILITATION PROTOCOL

A good rehabilitation program is the keystone to the progression of an injured athlete back to competition. The overall success of a program depends on realistic goals, patient compliance, and motivation.

Each athletic injury is unique, and as such a rehabilitation program should be tailored to the individual injury and level of competition. Some common goals are the reduction of pain and inflammation in the acute stage of the program so that a logical progession of training can occur. Most rehabilitation techniques for sports injuries are based on a functional program that attempts to prevent muscle atrophy; regain motion; and improve strength, power, and endurance.

With lower extremity injuries, the senior author uses a functional running program—which eliminates much of the conjecture that sometimes accompanies a decision to return the athlete to competition as expeditiously as possible. (See the Appendix on p. 255.) The running program can also be used as a measure of the athlete's progress toward return to play—so that when the program can be completed comfortably and in its entirety, the athlete can resume sport activities.

Through a comprehensive physical therapy program, the athlete may achieve the ultimate goal of any good functional program—to return the player to action as quickly and safely as possible.

## References

1. Ahmed AM, Burke DL: In vivo measurement of static pressure distribution in synovial joints. Part I: tibial surface of the knee, *J Biomech Eng* 105:201-209, 1983.
2. Anderson C, Odensten M, Gillquist J: Knee function after surgical and non-surgical treatment of acute rupture of the anterior cruciate ligament: a randomized study with long term follow-up period, *Clin Orthop* 264:255-263, 1991.
3. Anderson C, Odensten M, Good L, Gillquist J: Surgical or non-surgical treatment of anterior cruciate ligament: a randomized study with long term follow-up, *J Bone Joint Surg* 71A:965-974, 1989
4. Baratz ME, Fu JH, Mengato R: Meniscal tears: the effect of meniscectomy and of repair on intra-articular contact areas and stresses in the human knee, *Am J Sports Med* 14:270-275, 1986.
5. Barber FA, Stone RG: Meniscal repair: an arthroscopic technique, *J Bone Joint Surg* 67B:39-41, 1985.
6. Cassidy RE, Shaffer AJ: Repair of peripheral meniscal tears: a preliminary report, *Am J Sports Med* 9:209, 1981.
7. Clancy WG, Graf BK: Arthroscopic meniscal repair, *Orthopedics* 6:1125-1128, 1983.
8. Clancy WG, Ray JM, Zoltan DJ: Acute tears of the anterior cruciate ligament, *J Bone Joint Surg* 70A:1483-1488, 1988.
9. Clancy WG Jr, Shelbourne KD, Zoellner GB et al: Treatment of knee joint instability secondary to rupture of the posterior cruciate ligament: report of a new procedure, *J Bone Joint Surg* 65A:310-322, 1983.
10. Cox JS, Cordell LD: The degenerative effects of medial meniscal tears in dog's knees, *Clin Orthop* 125:236-242, 1977.
11. Cox JS, Nye CE, Schaeffer WW, Woodstein IJ: The degenerative effects of partial and total resection of the medial meniscus in dogs, *Clin Orthop* 109:178-183, 1975.
12. Cross MJ, Powell JF: Long-term follow-up of posterior cruciate ligament rupture: a study of 116 cases, *Am J Sports Med* 12:292-297, 1984.
13. Curwin S, Stanish WD: *Tendinitis: its etiology and treatment*, Lexington, Mass, 1984, Coollamare Press.
14. Dehaven KE: Decision making factors in the treatment of meniscal lesions, *Clin Orthop* 252:49-53, 1990.
15. Dehaven KE: Diagnosis of acute knee injuries with hemarthrosis, *Am J Sports Med* 8:901-914, 1980.
16. Dehaven KE: Meniscal repair in the athlete, *Clin Orthop* 198:31-35, 1985.
17. Dehaven KE: Peripheral meniscal repair: an alternative to meniscectomy, *J Bone Joint Surg* 63B:463, 1981.
18. Dehaven KE: Meniscectomy vs. repair: clinical experience. In Mow VC, Arnosky SP, Jackson DW, editors: *Knee meniscus: basic and clinical foundations*, New York, 1992, Raven Press.
19. Derscheid GL, Garrick JG: Medial collateral ligament injuries in football: non-operative management in Grade I and Grade II sprains, *Am J Sports Med* 9:365-368, 1981.

20. Fairbanks TJ: Knee joint changes after meniscectomy, *J Bone Joint Surg* 30B:664-670, 1948.
21. Fetto JF, Marshall JL: The natural history and diagnosis of anterior cruciate ligament insufficiency, *Clin Orthop* 147:29-38, 1980.
22. Fowler PJ, Messieh SS: Isolated posterior cruciate ligament injuries in athletes, *Am J Sports Med* 15:553-557, 1987.
23. Fowler PG, Regan WD: The patient with symptomatic chronic anterior cruciate ligament insufficiency: results of minimal arthroscopic surgery and rehabilitation, *Am J Sports Med* 15:321-325, 1987.
24. Fukubayashi T, Kurosawa H: The contact area and pressure distribution pattern of the knee: a study of normal and osteoarthritic knee joints, *Acta Orthop Scand* 51:871-880, 1980.
25. Giove TP, Miller SJ, Kent BE et al: Non-operative treatment of the torn anterior cruciate ligament, *J Bone Joint Surg* 65A:184-192, 1983.
26. Gollehon DL, Torzilli PA, Warren RF: The role of the posterolateral and cruciate ligaments in the stability of the human knee: a biomechanical study, *J Bone Joint Surg* 69A:233-242, 1987.
27. Grood ES, Stowers SF, Noyes FR: Limits of movement in the human knee: effect of sectioning the posterior cruciate ligament and posterolateral structures, *J Bone Joint Surg* 70A:88-97, 1988.
28. Hamberg P, Gillquist J, Lysholm J: Suture of new and old peripheral meniscal tears, *J Bone Joint Surg* 65A:193, 1983.
29. Hawkins RJ, Misamore GW, Merritt TR: Follow-up of acute non-operative isolated anterior cruciate ligament tears, *Am J Sports Med* 14:205-210, 1986.
30. Henning CE, Lynch MA, Clark JR: Vascularity for healing of meniscal repairs, *Arthroscopy* 3:13-18, 1987.
31. Hirshman HP, Daniel DM, Miyasaka K: The fate of unoperated knee ligament injuries. In Daniel DM, Akeson WH, O'Connor JJ, editors: *Knee ligaments: structure, function, injury, and repair*, New York, 1990, Raven Press.
32. Jackson RW: The torn ACL: natural history of untreated lesions and rationale for selective treatment. In Feagin JA, editor: *The crucial ligaments*, New York, 1988, Churchill Livingstone.
33. Jacobsen K: Osteoarthrosis following insufficiency of the cruciate ligaments in man: a clinical study, *Acta Orthop Scand* 48:520-526, 1977.
34. Johnson RJ, Kettlekamp DB, Clark W, Leaverton P: Factors affecting late results after meniscectomy, *J Bone Joint Surg* 56A:719-729, 1974.
35. Keller PM, Shelbourne KD, McCarroll JR et al: Nonoperatively treated isolated posterior cruciate ligament injuries, *Am J Sports Med* 21:132-136, 1993
36. Kennedy JC, Hawkins RJ, Willis RB et al: Tension studies of human knee ligaments, *J Bone Joint Surg* 58A:350, 1976.
37. Kettlekamp DB, Jacobs AW: The tibio-femoral contact area: determinations and implications, *J Bone Joint Surg* 54A:349-356, 1972.
38. Krause WR, Clemson MS, Pope MH et al: Mechanical changes in the knee after meniscectomy, *J Bone Joint Surg* 58A:599-604, 1976.
39. Levy M, Torzilli PA, Warren RF: The effect of medial meniscectomy on anterior-posterior motion of the knee, *J Bone Joint Surg* 64A:883-888, 1982.
40. Lynch MA, Henning CE, Glick KR: Knee joint surface changes: long term follow-up meniscus tear treatment in stable ACL reconstructions, *Clin Orthop* 172:148-153, 1983.
41. Marshall JL: Periarticular osteophytes: initiation and formation in the knee of the dog, *Clin Orthop* 62:37-47, 1969.

42. Marshall JL, Olsson SE: Instabililty of the knee: a long term experimental study in dogs, *J Bone Joint Surg* 53A:1561-1570, 1971.
43. Marshall JL, Rubin RM, Wang JB et al: The anterior cruciate ligament: the diagnosis and treatment of its injuries and their serious prognostic implications, *Orthop Rev* 7:35-46, 1978.
44. Marshall SC: Combined arthroscopic/open repair of meniscal injuries, *Contemp Orthop* 14:15-24, 1987.
45. McDaniel WJ Jr, Dameron TB Jr: The untreated anterior cruciate ligament rupture, *Clin Orthop* 172:158-163, 1983.
46. McDaniel WJ Jr, Dameron TB Jr: Untreated ruptures of the anterior cruciate ligament: a follow-up study, *J Bone Joint Surg* 62A:696-705, 1980.
47. McGinty JB, Geuss LF, Marvin RA: Partial or total meniscectomy? *J Bone Joint Surg* 59A:763-766, 1977.
48. Noyes FR, Bassett RW, Grood ES, Butler DL: Arthroscopy in acute traumatic hemarthrosis of the knee: incidence of anterior cruciate tears and other injuries, *J Bone Joint Surg* 62A:687-695, 1980.
49. Noyes FR, Matthews DS, Mooar PA, Grood ES: The symptomatic anterior cruciate deficient knee. Part II: the results of rehabilitation, activity modification, and counseling on functional disability, *J Bone Joint Surg* 65A:163-174, 1983.
50. Noyes FR et al: Advances in understanding knee ligament injury, repair and rehabilitation, *Med Sci Sports Exerc* 16:427-443, 1984.
51. O'Donoghue DH: Surgical treatment of fresh injuries to the major ligaments of the knee, *J Bone Joint Surg* 37A:1-13, 1955.
52. Parolie JM, Bergfeld JA: Long-term results of non-operative treatment of isolated posterior cruciate ligament injuries in the athlete, *Am J Sports Med* 14:35-38, 1986.
53. Satku K, Kumar VP, Ngoi SS: Anterior cruciate ligament injuries. To counsel or to operate? *J Bone Joint Surg* 68B:458-461, 1986.
54. Sherman MF, Warren RF, Marshall JL et al: A clinical and radiographic analysis of 127 anterior cruciate insufficient knees, *Clin Orthop* 227:229-237, 1988.
55. Tapper EM, Hoover NW: Late results after meniscectomy, *J Bone Joint Surg* 51A:517-526, 1969.
56. Torg JS, Barton TM, Pavlov H et al: Natural history of the posterior cruciate ligament-deficient knee, *Clin Orthop* 246:208-216, 1989.
57. Trickey EL: Rupture of the posterior cruciate ligament of the knee, *J Bone Joint Surg* 50B:334-341, 1968.
58. Walla DJ, Albright JP, McAuley E et al: Hamstring control and the unstable anterior cruciate ligament deficient knee, *Am J Sports Med* 13:34-39, 1985.
59. Warner JP, Warren RF, Cooper DE: Management of anterior cruciate ligament injuries, *Instr Course Lect* 40:219-232, 1990.
60. Warren RF, Marshall JL: Injuries of the anterior cruciate and medial collateral ligaments of the knee, *Clin Orthop* 136:191, 1978.
61. Zairns B, Adams M: Medical progress: knee injuries in sports, *N Engl J Med* 318:950-961, 1988.

# Chapter 14

# Injuries to the leg and ankle

Michael J. Kaplan
William G. Clancy, Jr.
James R. Andrews

The on-field evaluation of leg and ankle injuries includes a multitude of injury patterns. Athletic competition, and field sport in particular, presents a high risk for lower extremity trauma. Football, soccer, field hockey, lacrosse, and other contact sports are typically implicated in the more acute injuries; baseball, tennis, and track and field are more characteristically associated with overuse types of phenomena. Nonetheless, any of the injuries reflected in the myriad of subheadings that follow can occur as a result of the high exertional activities that are the mainstay of stop, start, jump, and change-of-direction maneuvers of outdoor sports.

## FRACTURE AND FRACTURE DISLOCATION

### CLOSED INJURIES

Fracture and fracture dislocation can result from any mechanism wherein sufficient energy is transmitted to the bone and/or joint and causes failure of the type I or type II collagen bundles, respectively. Bone is strongest in compression, so bending, rotational, and sheer stresses are typically responsible for breaks. Ligament, tendon, capsule, and muscle are strongest in tension, and their yield points are also directly dependent on the direction of load. All of these tissue types demonstrate, to different degrees, viscoelastic properties (i.e., their elastic modulus and critical point of energy absorption before failure are rate dependent). Bone, for instance, fractures at less force application with slower force transmission. Moreover, fracture patterns reflect the impact or load itself. Spiral or long fractures are typically low-energy injuries, whereas transverse fractures are more often related to high impact. Comminution, or multiple fragmentation, is associated with exceedingly high loads.

Athletes who suffer fractures frequently recall a "snap" or "crack" with an instantaneous onset of pain and inability to bear weight. Pain can be diffuse in nature, but focal intensity localizes bony injury. Objective findings are largely dependent on accompanying soft tissue injury—with the degree of swelling, ecchymosis, and palpation tenderness relative to underlying bony disruption. Painful active and passive range of motion of joints above and below the injury are further clues to the extent of the trauma. Acute gross deformity in limb alignment, contour, or color suggests the possibility of fracture and must be treated as such until otherwise confirmed by off-field evaluation (including x-ray).

Initial splinting, limb support, elevation, and light cryocompression ready an injured athlete for transport off the field. Athletes with lower leg injuries are best transferred out of the playing terrain by a stretcher or cart to an ambulance, and then to a medical facility. Athletic gear and equipment should be left in place except for obviously aggravating paraphernalia. No one with an injury suspected of being a fracture and/or dislocation should be observed on the sideline or allowed to return to play without physician clearance. When there is a question about whether an injury is an ankle ligament sprain (versus an ankle fracture), and particularly when there is no ligamentous laxity on examination, a fracture should be suspected if the athlete cannot jump up and down on the extremity.

## OPEN INJURIES

Open fractures and/or dislocations represent a surgical emergency and necessitate urgent attention and transport to a hospital. Field measures include those already mentioned for closed injuries, with the addition of a sterile dressing covering exposed tissue. Bleeding sites are tamponaded by direct pressure with a sterile gauze or pad, with no use of a constricting bandage or tourniquet. Description of field conditions and environmental toxins should be transmitted with the alerting call to the designated treating medical professional.

## LACERATIONS AND ABRASIONS

Soft tissue wounds can occur anywhere, as the leg and ankle are frequently associated with high-energy and contact sports. Linear cuts usually result from a penetration or sheer contact force from a sharp object. Stellate lacerations, tissue avulsions, and dermal abrasions result from blunt impact or wide-contact sheer transmission energies.

Diagnosis is made easily with inspection and palpation. One must be sure to recognize underlying soft tissue and bony injury and not be simply concerned with hemorrhage and skin debris. Wound evaluation should be done off the field once dressings have been applied and bleeding tamponaded. Blunt pressure by hand or bandage at oozing sites usually suffices. Again, no tourniquets or tourniquet-effect dressings are to be used. After proper cleaning with antibiotic solution, sterile evaluation of the wound is carried out. Local anesthetics can be used to close clean wounds with even and easily opposable edges. Large stellate or dirty wounds should be left open after cleaning (for healing by secondary intention) but obviously deserve physician evaluation. Return to play is dictated by the size of the wound and the degree and stability of its healing. Incompletely healed tissue must be adequately protected with dressings and pads, and there must be a minimum of discomfort with range of motion of the joints above and below so as not to limit performance. Antibiotic coverage with topical and systemic medicines is dictated by specific circumstances.

## FIBULAR HEAD SUBLUXATION OR DISLOCATION

Acute and chronic instability of the fibular head is a relatively uncommon injury. The most common presentation is that of an anterior lateral translation relative to the knee followed by a posterior medial dislocation. Superior translations are almost always associated with fibular fracture. The mechanism of injury typically involves an inversion and plantar flexion of the foot with tension of the peroneal muscle group and long extensors of the foot.[1] Violent contraction of these muscles can pull the fibula forward when the knee is in flexion and the biceps and fibulocollateral ligament are relaxed.

Patients typically have acute pain over the proximal tibia-fibula joint (Fig. 14-1). Active flexion and extension of the ankle with concomitant inversion and eversion are usually painful and can occasionally transmit paresthesias from the peroneal nerve.[1] If swelling is minimal, an obvious prominence of the fibula can be appreciated with associated tenderness to palpation and attempted reduction. The proximal fibular instability can usually be appreciated with an anteroposterior translation force by grasping the fibula between the thumb and index finger. X-ray and fluoroscopy can be helpful to solidify the diagnosis.

Acute treatment off the field would include closed reduction, usually with some type of anesthetic. A short period of knee immobilization and the minimization of weight-bearing are appropriate until the patient is pain-free. Rehabilitation includes a quadriceps and hamstring strengthening program, with return to play predicated on complete return of range of motion, resolution of tenderness to palpation, and at least an 85% return of strength relative to the contralateral limb. A counterforce brace and/or taping may be helpful in the early stages.

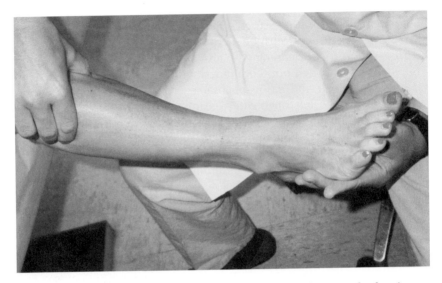

**Fig. 14-1.** Fibular head instability produces pain with palpation. The foot is supported with 15 degree flexion at the knee.

## MEDIAL GASTROCNEMIUS TEAR (TENNIS LEG)

This is a relatively common injury, most frequently seen among athletes in their late 20s and 30s. This injury typically presents in the poorly conditioned individual and is frequently thought to be the result of improper or insufficient stretching. Over-stretching of this two-joint–spanning muscle results from forced ankle dorsiflexion with an extended knee. Patients relate a sudden onset of pain in the calf while running or with a sudden stop, cut, or landing. The swelling and pain increase over a 24- to 48-hour period as a result of hemorrhage and increased tissue permeability. Objective findings include tenderness and an occasional palpable defect at the musculotendinous junction of the medial head of the gastrocnemius (Fig. 14-2). Passive dorsiflexion beyond neutral with the knee in extension elicits pain, and patients frequently have difficulty with push-off during the initial postinjury period. The differential diagnosis must include thrombophlebitis, phlebothrombosis, and posterior compartment syndrome.[1]

Initial treatment consists of ice, elevation, a supportive wrap, and a few days of no weight bearing.[1] Early range of motion of the ankle is begun with an active and active-assisted regimen. Nonsteroidal anti-inflammatory drugs can be helpful once the bleeding has ceased (at least 48 hours after injury). A passive stretching program within the limits of pain is initiated by the end of the first week and (along with either a heel lift or a walking boot orthotic [Fig. 14-3]) can be used for symptomatic

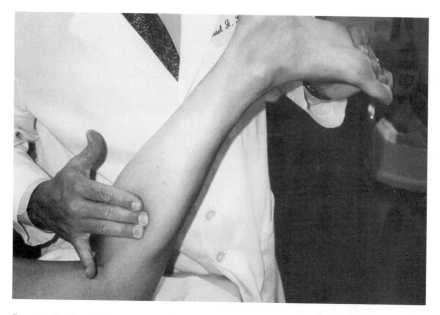

**Fig. 14-2.** Tennis leg, or a medial gastrocnemius tear, is tender at the musculo-tendinous junction. Occasionally hemorrhage and a defect are appreciated.

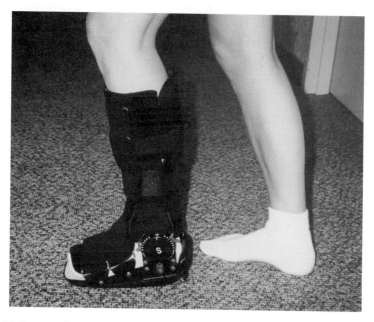

**Fig. 14-3.** A walking boot orthotic controls plantar flexion stress with a rocker bottom sole.

relief for the initial 2 or 3 weeks. A strengthening program should be initiated by 2 weeks postinjury, with a goal of return to sport by 5 or 6 weeks postinjury—depending on the clinical exam and strength quotient. A full range of motion, 80% plantar flexion strength relative to the contralateral leg, and a pain-free exam to deep palpation of the medial gastrocnemius must be present before full performance is to be expected.

## POPLITEAL ARTERY ENTRAPMENT

Ischemic types of symptoms, such as achiness and pain associated with activity but relieved with rest, must raise the suspicion for a vascular-compromising lesion. This rare phenomenon can be best demonstrated with active plantar flexion and passive hyperdorsiflexion of an affected individual's leg.[1] Doppler examination is frequently insufficient; arteriogram is necessary to establish the diagnosis and should be used when sufficient clinical suspicion is raised. Arterial occlusion is usually at the level of the medial gastrocnemius origin, and flow is mechanically impeded by a fascial or scar band. When diagnosis is confirmed, the treatment is surgical release with occasional fasciotomy. Conservative measures are ineffective in relieving symptoms. Return to play is predicated on healing of the wound, pain-free gradual return to exercise, and functional goal attainment. Consultation with a vascular surgeon is essential.

## MEDIAL TIBIAL STRESS SYNDROME

Medial tibial stress syndrome encompasses several discrete injury patterns. They are grouped together because of their common presentation of medial or anterior leg pain that accompanies overuse activities of high axial impact. Stress or fatigue fractures of the tibia are typically characterized by focal tenderness to palpation and varus-valgus stress of the long bone (Fig. 14-4). Periostitis; insertional tendinitis of the soleus and posterior tibialis (shin splints); compartmental fasciitis; muscle herniation; and contusion of bone and soft tissue are often difficult to distinguish in the acute setting. Close attention to the area of maximum sensitivity and inspection of the area can often help in the differential diagnosis. Active and passive range of motion of the ankle and knee will usually elicit pain from injuries to the soft tissues. Paramount to an accurate assessment is the history of onset of pain and the mechanism of injury.

Patients have activity-induced, dull, achy pain of the leg that usually results from an increase in duration or intensity of running. If untreated,

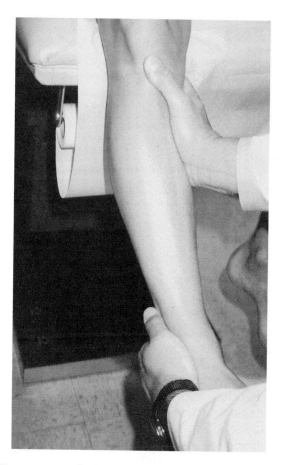

**Fig. 14-4.** Varus stress to the leg elicits pain with a stress or fatigue fracture.

it can progress to severe, disabling pain. Thought to be a result of fasciitis or periostitis at the tibial insertion of the soleus and posterior tibialis, the patient with medial stress syndrome is typically tender to palpation at the posterior medial ridge of the middle and distal tibia. Resisted plantar flexion of the foot can elicit pain. The normal foot pronation that occurs with heel strike puts an eccentric stress on the soleus muscle. Increased pronation of the foot may predispose an individual to increased soleus stress and is associated with the development of overuse syndromes in the lower extremities.[10] The initial treatment for this overuse type of injury is active rest. Athletes are advised to avoid running and exercises that exacerbate their symptoms. Instead, we promote conditioning and encourage involvement in exercises such as swimming and biking. These and other low-impact exercises are the mainstay of treatment while allowing sufficient time for healing. Correction of lower limb alignment via orthotics is also essential. Stretching tight heel cords and using ultrasound, nonsteroidal antiinflammatory medicines, cryotherapy, and whirlpool all may be beneficial in the early stages.

Return to play after a medial stress syndrome is dictated by the ability of the athlete to perform agility and endurance drills at 85% strength relative to the preinjury or contralateral limb status. Full range of motion and a painless exam are mandatory. In general, at least 1 to 2 weeks of active rest are necessary to quiet the acute inflammatory condition before a trial return-to-play period. It is not unusual for it to take up to 6 weeks for full return, and recurrences are relatively common. Surgical release of the fascial envelope insertion is reserved for those few recalcitrant cases.

## STRESS FRACTURES

Stress fractures can occur anywhere in the lower extremity, with the most common site being the proximal or distal tibia. Frequently associated with running on hard surfaces, stress fractures are thought to result from repetitive stress and bone resorption occurring more rapidly than bone proliferation. There are two general theories for the cause of a tibial stress fracture: the first proposes muscle fatigue[17] and the second refers to muscle overpowerment.[16] Symptoms are usually gradual in onset (over weeks) following a change in training. Patients complain of focal pain throughout their exercise and often can point to the fatigue fracture. Consideration of underlying metabolic abnormality secondary to either immobilization, amenorrhea, or nutritional deficiency is important to rule out a metabolic, neurologic, or hormonal cause of the stress injury. Sport activities involving repetitive axial impact—such as running, gymnastics, or dancing—are common causes of stress fractures about the ankle (i.e., the medial or lateral malleolus). There is usually mild swelling and point tenderness in these regions as well. Percussion over the bone itself can cause pain and associated erythema and warmth; occasional tibia vara or anterior bowing may be evident. Radiographic confirmation by plain film x-rays typically takes at least 3 to 5 weeks before callus is apparent. Bone scans may be positive as soon as 3 days after injury.

The treatment of stress injuries to the lower extremity primarily involves active or relative rest. Nonsteroidals, electrical stimulation, correction of the biomechanical or medical problem, and modification in the training and exercise program are the mainstays of treatment. It is important to maintain an athlete's aerobic capacity and leg strength and to have him or her begin weight bearing with an orthotic or supports as tolerated. A walking boot or air cast is a very helpful supplement and may be instrumental in expediting an athlete's progress with gait training and resumption of sport activity. Nonunion or displacement of a fracture warrants treatment with open reduction and internal fixation.

Return to play is usually allowed when the patient is no longer painful to palpation around the injured area. Mature callus is generally apparent on a plain film x-ray and typically takes at least 6 to 8 weeks from the onset of pain to form. Return to competition should be based on a gentle and pain-free return to activity, with satisfaction of functional goals such as those outlined in the running program. (See the Appendix on p. 255.)

## CHRONIC COMPARTMENT SYNDROME

A compartment syndrome is defined as an increased pressure in a closed fibroosseous space that reduces blood flow and tissue perfusion. The diagnosis of an acute compartment syndrome is usually easily apparent because of the severe pain, acute swelling, and compartment tenseness that accompanies severe trauma to soft tissue and bone. This surgical emergency, which presents most commonly in the lower leg, necessitates emergency compartment pressure measurements after expeditious transfer to a hospital facility. The diagnosis of a chronic exertional compartment syndrome, which is the type most often found in athletes, is less readily recognized. It nonetheless represents a significant lower extremity injury pattern, necessitating evaluation and often decompression of the involved compartment via fasciotomy. The athlete usually has exercise-induced calf or leg pain that resolves with rest. It usually affects an athlete who runs long distances or has a recent increase in duration or intensity of training. The athlete typically has a tense or tight calf muscle compartment with pain on passive range of motion of the ankle. Exercise can increase muscle volume or weight by up to 20%.[5] The pathophysiology of an increased compartment volume and muscle swelling is thought to be secondary to an increase in capillary permeability with resultant edema and restricted venous and lymphatic outflow of tissue fluids.[11] Acute ischemia and hemorrhage from muscle tearing are likewise potential causal factors. Any of the four leg compartments, most often the anterior, can be subject to substantial pressure increase with strenuous exercise. Transient tingling or numbness (paresthesias) can accompany the symptoms of intense pain. Athletes seeking medical attention complain of a predictable onset of symptoms with a causal relationship to specific athletic events, and their time to relief with rest is referable to the severity of their syndrome. Bilaterality, to some extent, can be seen in up to 90% of patients.

Diagnosis is confirmed with knowledge of the injury's history—after clinical exam demonstrates pain with passive motion or stretching of the muscle compartments; increased calf girth or circumference; decreased sensation to the first web space of the foot; and, most importantly, pressure compartment measurements before and after exercise. Slit catheter or striker instrumented pressure measurements made 1 and 5 minutes after exercise with elevations of greater than 30 and 20 mm Hg, respectively, are diagnostic.[5] Conservative measures are rarely helpful except for activity modification measures. Rather, surgical release of the compartment via fasciotomy is the mainstay of treatment for chronic compartment syndrome and is highly successful in relieving symptoms.[14] Nevertheless, in addition to the potential for infection and delayed wound healing, fasciotomy is also thought to decrease its enveloping muscle's strength by up to 15%.

When making the diagnosis of chronic compartment syndrome, one must always be cognizant of the differential diagnosis, including stress fracture, posterior tibial tendinitis, periostitis, fascial defects, medial gastrocnemius tears, and vascular occlusion–induced ischemia.

## ACHILLES TENDON INJURIES

### ACHILLES TENDON TEAR

Rupture of the Achilles tendon typically results from an abrupt and substantial dorsiflexion load to the foot and leg. Landing on one's foot or a quick take-off plantar flexion acceleration accounts for the majority of the mechanisms responsible for Achilles tears. Athletes report a "pop" or "snap" with loss of plantar flexion strength and difficulty bearing weight. The differential diagnosis includes partial tearing, plantaris rupture, and medial gastrocnemius tearing.

Physical examination reveals exquisite tenderness about the musculotendinous junction of the gastrocnemius soleus complex, with ecchymosis and swelling. Often, an examiner can appreciate a palpable defect and definitive weakness of active plantar flexion. A positive Thompson test (squeezing the gastrocnemius) (Fig. 14-5) at 90 degrees of knee flexion should elicit no or little foot plantar flexion. This, like all exams, should be done with comparison to the contralateral, uninjured extremity. The athlete suffering this injury is immediately removed from play for icing and gentle compressive dressing. Definitive treatment with casting rather than surgery continues to be debated: the advocates for a surgical correction contend that surgery yields better strength and mobility, with a decreased rerupture rate, whereas the conservative, or nonoperative, proponents maintain that their approach results in a decreased morbidity, without the prospect of wound healing problems or infection.[9]

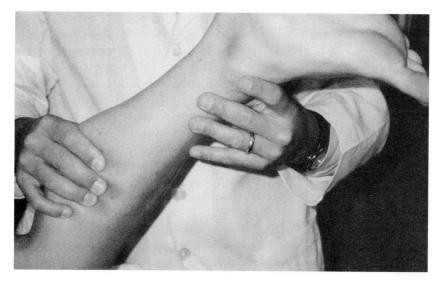

**Fig. 14–5.** A positive Thompson test reveals no plantar flexion of the foot with calf compression (knee is flexed).

## ACHILLES TENDINITIS AND TENOSYNOVITIS

Achilles tendinitis refers to an inflammatory condition of the tendon itself. Tenosynovitis and peritendinitis are terms referring to inflammation of the tendon sheath or cover that lines the tendon, without necessarily involving the tendon itself. Tendinosis refers to an intrasubstance degeneration or focal necrosis of tendon. Although each of these three entities is a distinct pathology deserving separate consideration, in this section we include their common presentations and on-field treatment regimens as a whole. Suffice it to say that a partial rupture or nonviable collagen tissue within the tendon can be the result of an acute injury or the sequela of repetitive microtrauma with prolonged inflammation.

Underlying factors that are responsible for inflammation about the Achilles tendon include excessive foot pronation; chronic Achilles tendon contracture; stiff footwear; and overweight, unconditioned athletes—all of which contribute to the increased work at the muscle-tendon complex. Physical examination includes findings of pain and swelling about the area of tendon injury, with pain on active and passive stretch. A bulbous focal lesion should make one suspect tearing or tendinosis (Fig. 14-6), whereas more diffuse, fusiform swelling is typical of peritendinitis.

Initial treatment is focused on decreasing inflammation with minimization of tendon excursion, occasionally necessitating immobilization in a walking boot or cast. Ice, ultrasound, and other modalities can be helpful. The use of a heel lift via a $\frac{1}{2}$-cm shoe insert oftentimes can

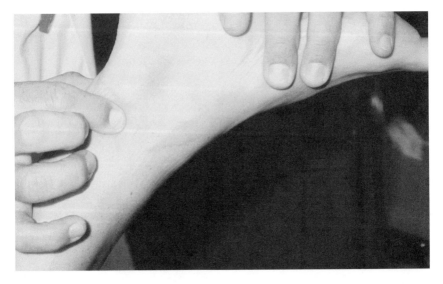

**Fig. 14-6.** The Achilles tendon is palpated to assess for bulbous or fusiform swelling. Tenderness is elicited with this maneuver if injury is present.

normalize gait and make athletes considerably more comfortable. After the acute inflammatory phase has resolved, stretching of the musculotendinous complex is important. The use of a heel lift to decrease tendon excursion and minimize dorsiflexion strain should continue for at least several weeks after symptoms subside. Magnetic resonance imaging (MRI) is helpful to determine if there is intratendinous degeneration and to identify tendon tears that may be an indication for surgical debridement (should the lesions be recalcitrant to the above conservative measures). Once again, return to sport is dictated by fulfilling functional criteria that would include completion of a running program. (See the Appendix on p. 255.)

## ANKLE SPRAIN

### LATERAL SPRAIN

The majority of ankle sprains occur during plantar flexion, adduction, and inversion.[13] It is in this position that the anterior talofibular ligament (ATFL) is most taut and at risk for injury. The calcaneofibular ligament (CFL) primarily restrains inversion of the calcaneus with respect to the fibula. Its primary role is in a dorsiflexed ankle position. Typically the ATFL is injured first; followed by the CFL; and, finally, if the force is violent enough, the posterior fibular ligament (PTFL) is torn. Renstrom contends that "In dorsiflexion, a syndesmosis rupture (anterior and posterior inferior tibial fibular ligament with the interosseous membrane) is most likely to occur."[12] According to Brostrum, the ATFL was solely involved in 65% of the sprains, with the CFL included in another 20% of cases.[3] The syndesmosis was involved in 10% of cases, and the deltoid or medial ligaments were involved 3% of the time.[3]

Ankle sprains have traditionally been classified into one of three grades. A grade I injury is characterized by stretching of the ligament with only microscopic tearing. These are mild injuries with minimal swelling or tenderness. Grade II ligament sprains infer a partial tear of the tissue with substantial swelling, ecchymosis, and tenderness. Grade III tears are complete ligament ruptures that are often accompanied by the perception of a "pop" or "snap" by the patient at injury. These severe injuries have pronounced swelling, ecchymosis, and pain to palpation.

The on-field evaluation of an athlete complaining of ankle pain must include taking a history of any previous ankle injury and treatments. The number and degree of sprains are relevant to a patient's instability pattern. The mechanism of injury is also crucial in confirming the diagnosis. The sensation of tearing or an audible "snap" and the inability to bear weight, along with the duration between insult and symptoms, are directly related to the magnitude of the injury.

An appreciation of the anatomy through a deliberate and repeatable sequence in the exam is essential. Palpation of specific structures to elicit pain helps in recognizing the site and degree of trauma. Swelling, ecchymosis, and subtle anatomic distortions relative to the contralateral leg help confirm a diagnosis. Palpation to identify a gap or a prominence in tissue planes, along with an inspection of the joints above and below the area of complaint, is also included. We begin examining the apparently uninvolved region and then proceed lastly to the area of obvious derangement. Assessment of the contralateral normal ankle to appreciate a patient's baseline stability and anatomic configurations is fundamental. Active and passive range of motion parameters are recorded before stress testing of the ankle. The predictive capabilities of the anterior drawer and talar tilt tests are more valuable immediately after injury, before pronounced edema and resultant pain ensue.

The anterior drawer test (Fig. 14-7) is performed by firmly grasping the patient's heel (examiner's right hand to patient's right heel) with one hand and providing an anterior force while stabilizing the patient's distal leg with the other hand using a posterior buttress. The exam is best performed with the patient sitting with the knee flexed 90 degrees to relax the gastrocnemius muscle complex. The ankle joint is optimally at neutral or slight plantar flexion. Only gross anterior displacement relative to the contralateral ankle is reliably detectable, inferring

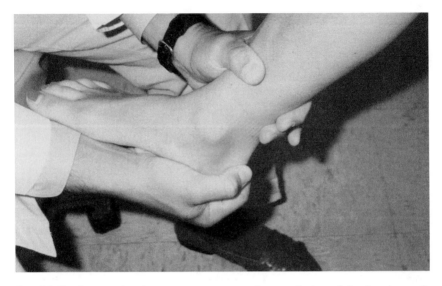

**Fig. 14-7.** The anterior drawer test measures the translation of the foot beneath the leg and the competence of the anterior talofibular ligament (ATFL).

significant ankle laxity. Although the ATFL is commonly thought to be the ligament responsible for limiting anterior translation, "it is not known to what extent the different ankle ligaments are involved during this test and to what extent anterior talar displacement occurs in the talocrural joint and in the subtalar joints."[12] The talar tilt test is meant to measure the integrity of the calcaneal fibular ligament (Fig. 14-8). Examined in neutral or slight dorsiflexion of the ankle, the heel is inverted with a varus stress while the distal leg is held firm. Talar tilt refers to the lateral opening of the ankle at the tibiotalar joint. Again, this test is of questionable reliability except in the most flagrant of instability patterns. Guarding because of pain-induced muscular resistance can be minimized by local injection but is discouraged except in the office setting.

The differential diagnosis for lateral ankle sprain injury is substantial. Many of the potential injury patterns are commonly sustained by athletes. All ankle and lower leg injuries that are accompanied by severe pain, swelling, ecchymosis, loss of motion, functional disability, or palpable defect are obligatorily evaluated by radiograph and oftentimes ancillary objective tests (depending on the circumstance). It is the responsibility of the sideline or treating health personnel to rule out serious injury before reinstatement of activity or even the rehabilitative process. The differential diagnosis for lateral ankle sprains includes bony fractures of the lateral, medial, and posterior malleolus, proximal fibula, lateral or

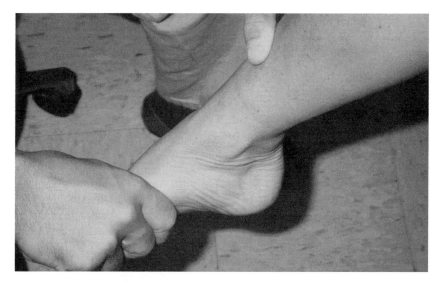

**Fig. 14-8.** The talar tilt test uses varus stress to assess instability of the calcaneo-fibular ligament (CFL).

posterior process of the talus, anterior process of the calcaneus, fifth metatarsal, navicular, and other tarsal bones. Any of these fractures can accompany an injury pattern consistent with the mechanism and clinical exam of ankle inversion trauma. Osteochondral fractures of the talar dome or tibial plafond can also coexist with an ankle sprain and significantly alter the natural history of a patient's course. Midfoot sprains, peroneal tendon subluxations or dislocations, and ankle tendon tears or inflammation are also potential mimickers of a "simple" ankle sprain. Finally, medial ankle or deltoid ligament sprains and syndesmosis tearing are ankle injuries that need to be recognized and are discussed separately later.

## TREATMENT

After an ankle sprain is diagnosed, a clinical grading of the ligament damage helps dictate the treatment plan. Initial management for all types begins with rest, ice, compression, and elevation (RICE). These measures are used immediately (on the sideline). Immobilization and non–weight-bearing status are minimized in grade I and II injuries and the duration of these measures is best dictated by functional status and clinical exam parameters. The rationale for RICE therapy is to minimize hemorrhage, edema, inflammation, and pain. Temporary immobilization of the injured structure is thought prudent to foster initial scar formation via type II collagen proliferation.[8] The maturation of scar (approximately 3 weeks after injury) to well-oriented collagen fibers is enhanced by controlled stretching of muscles and movement of the joint.[12] Prolonged immobilization causes tissue atrophy,[8] whereas exercise increases the mechanical and structural properties of the ligaments.[18] After 4 to 6 weeks, the collagen fibers begin to assume strength characteristics that enable them to assume almost normal stress. Final remodeling of the soft tissue is not complete before 6 to 8 months.

The first treatment program, along with RICE therapy, includes a short protection period of 1 to 3 weeks. Taping or a semirigid orthosis with early controlled mobilization in a frontal plane that does not stretch the ligament is important. Weight bearing within pain limits is immediately begun. By 2 to 3 weeks after the injury, mobilization to include inversion and eversion exercises is begun along with stationary biking and stretching of the Achilles tendon. A bongo board (tilt board) for proprioception is implemented at 4 to 8 weeks postinjury. A balance and neuromuscular control program[6] maximizing peroneal muscle strength and general muscular strengthening via a Theraband cord for eccentric training is essential. A running program beginning with isokinetic exercises is used toward a goal of strength, power, and endurance. (See the Appendix on p. 255.) Supportive treatments to promote recovery include ultrasound, temperature-controlled baths, and shortwave therapy. Dynamic or interference current therapy, electrogalvanic stimulation, and cryotherapy have proven effective in trials.[7] Nonsteroidal antiinflammatory medicines are effective early on as well.[4] Joint aspiration with corticosteroid injection appears to be helpful but cannot be recommended at this time. Ultimately, 10% of patients with lateral ligament injury have chronic symptoms (i.e., inflammation, stiffness, swelling, pain and weakness, and the feeling of "giving way").

It is important to note that ankle taping, although effective initially, loses up to 50% of its original support after 10 minutes of exercise.[13] Ankle braces (Fig. 14-9) are more effective prophylactically than taping for preventing injury.[15] Taping necessitates an underwrap or skin lubricant and is technique-dependent.

Our general rule for return to play includes full active and passive range of motion. Patients must be able to walk, run, hop, and do change-of-direction sport activities without pain or limping in accordance with our running program. (See the Appendix on p. 255.) We aim for an 85% return of strength compared with the contralateral ankle and require athletes to perform a full sprint with minimal to no loss of speed before return to competition.

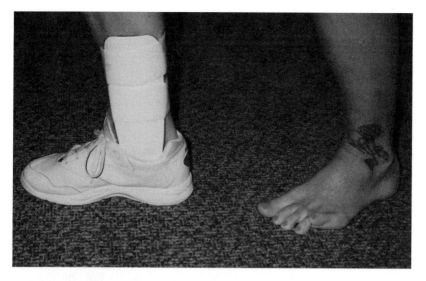

**Fig. 14-9.** A plastic commercial ankle brace allows the athlete to wear normal footgear and protects against varus and valgus stress.

## MEDIAL ANKLE INJURY OR DELTOID INJURY

The tibial calcaneal and tibial navicular ligaments support the talocrural and subtalar joints. The deep tibiotalar ligaments are more important for ankle stability and support only the talocrural joint. Only 3% of ankle sprains are reported to involve the medial side exclusively.[3] Typically injured with either pronation-abduction, pronation-external rotation, or supination-external rotation mechanisms, these ligament injuries can be either midsubstance or result in avulsion of bone from the medial malleolus or talus.[12] The differential diagnosis includes syndesmosis injury with or without fracture, in addition to the myriad of other injury patterns previously described in the lateral ankle sprain segment. Pain, swelling, and tenderness are primarily medially located, and a valgus eversion test is performed with comparison to the other ankle. Like lateral ligament injuries, partial tears are cared for with conservative measures much like the type I and type II injuries previously mentioned. There is no consensus on the treatment of complete, or grade III, tears of the deltoid ligament. Except for those injuries associated with instability or other concomitant tissue damage, the majority of deltoid ligament injuries are cared for with a conservative regimen, much like injuries in the lateral ankle. Also, just as for lateral ligament injuries, late reconstructive procedures for residual instability offer results comparable with acute repairs and therefore support the rationale for an initial nonoperative approach.

## TIBIOFIBULAR SYNDESMOSIS TEAR

The anterior and posterior tibiofibular ligaments and interosseous membranes account for approximately 10% of ankle injuries.[12] The highest incidence of this injury occurs in football, with a dorsiflexion and external rotation mechanism. Diastasis of the syndesmosis, with partial or complete rupture of the syndesmosis ligament complex, occurs. An isolated rupture of the soft tissue without fracture is rare but can occur. Plain x-rays with mortise measurements and bone scan are objective correlates (Figs. 14-10 and 14-11). The deltoid is commonly injured along with syndesmosis tearing and is more commonly associated with medial and/or posterior malleolar fractures.

On physical examination, pain and tenderness can be elicited at the anterior aspect of the ankle (Fig. 14-12). External rotation of the foot is exquisitely painful (Fig. 14-13). A squeeze test of the tibia and fibula at the midleg (Fig. 14-14)—along with a positive cotton test for gripping of the calcaneus, with medial and lateral rocking while holding the distal leg—is also used. Athletes are unable to bear weight with significant syndesmosis tearing, and they must be removed from play. This sometimes

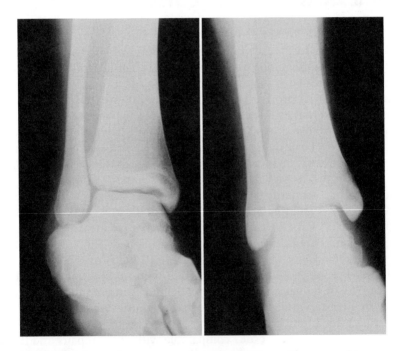

**Fig. 14-10.** Mortise and anteroposterior x-rays of the ankle are used to measure the interspace between the medial malleolus and the lateral malleolus.

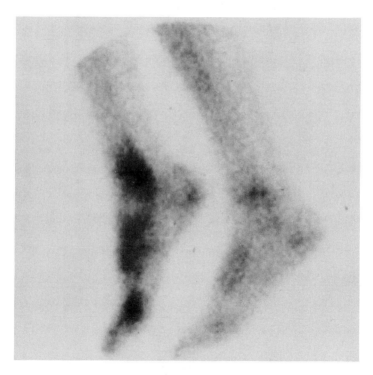

**Fig. 14-11.** A bone scan can objectively testify to soft tissue and bony injury.

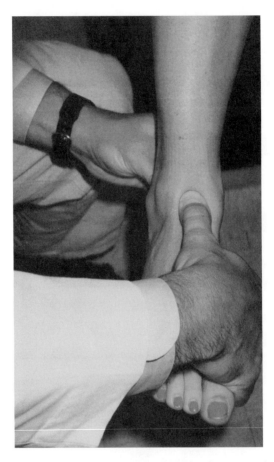

**Fig. 14-12.** Palpation of the anterior ankle elicits tenderness with anteroinferior tibiofibular ligament tearing.

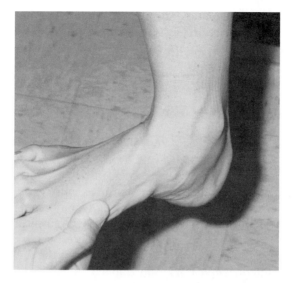

**Fig. 14-13.** Passive external rotation of the ankle stresses the tibiofibular syndesmosis.

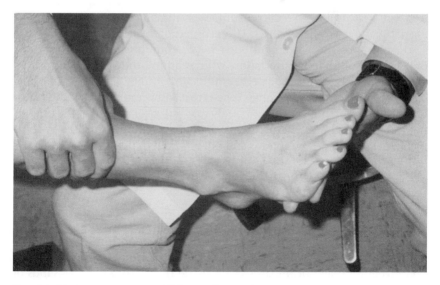

**Fig. 14-14.** Firm squeezing of the midleg with pressure on the fibula and tibia elicits pain with syndesmosis tearing.

subtle sprain complex typically necessitates a prolonged recovery period, but treatment and return to play criteria follow along the same lines as the previously discussed lateral ligament injuries. Nonetheless, a distinction must be made, as syndesmosis widening confirmed by an x-ray may necessitate operative correction; and certainly the recovery period and downtime from sport are considerably longer.

## NERVE COMPRESSION SYNDROMES

The deep peroneal, superficial peroneal, sural, and posterior tibial nerves can all be irritated or entrapped and exhibit the myriad of symptoms included in ankle and leg injuries. Ankle joint instability, soft tissue and bony impingement, chronic compartment syndromes, muscle herniations, and simple contusions can all elicit symptoms of nerve compression.[2] Symptoms such as burning pain and numbness should raise the suspicion that an athlete has a nerve compression phenomenon. Anterior tarsal tunnel syndrome or compression of the deep peroneal nerve is the most common of these entities, and the nerve is typically trapped under the inferior extensor retinaculum.[2] The superficial peroneal nerve is typically entrapped as it pierces the deep fascia entering the lateral compartment of the leg 10 to 12 cm above the tip of the lateral malleolus.[2] Sural nerve entrapment is most frequently secondary to recurrent ankle sprains, and it is marked by shooting pains and paresthesias to the lateral aspect of the heel and foot.

Diagnosis of the aforementioned nerve compression syndromes can only be made with full appreciation of the anatomy and by eliciting positive Tinel's signs with confirming nerve conduction studies. Frequently, an athlete with one of these syndromes who is recalcitrant to change footwear or use stabilizing orthotics will ultimately need surgical release of the offending scar band or tissue.[2] Return to play in these instances is dictated by complete amelioration of symptoms and full attainment of functional goals.

## RUNNING INJURIES

Many of the already mentioned discrete injury patterns result from the repetitive stress placed on the lower extremities from running. The vertical or ground reaction force at midstance ranges from $1\frac{1}{2}$ to 5 times the body weight.[11] Significant stresses on tissue result from the thousands of foot contacts associated with running. A slight biomechanical abnormality or joint alteration can profoundly upset tissue loads. Renstrom separates causes into extrinsic and intrinsic categories. He reports that 60% to 80% of running injuries are the result of extrinsic factors.[11] Most commonly, errors in training are at fault. Structural abnormalities account for the majority of the intrinsic factors, which include cavus feet, leg length discrepancies, joint contracture, and poor muscle conditioning.[11] Muscle weakness is known to predispose a joint to instability and decreased shock absorption; likewise, neuromuscular coordination is integral to the proprioception necessary for appropriate joint mechanics.[11]

An injury to the soft tissues that is associated with running typically heals with scar tissue that has an elasticity different from virgin tissue. Risk of re-injury increases with the fibrosis and adhesions that are characteristic of joint complexes that have sustained multiple injuries. Moreover, joint instability and effusion result in reflex inhibition and subsequent atrophy of muscle, with a compensatory increase in joint and soft tissue stresses. Renstrom expounds on the need to evaluate the entire kinetic chain of the lower extremity as a series of mobile segments and linkages that allow forward propulsion through gait.[11] An appreciation of an athlete's running mileage, training conditions, modification in techniques, shoewear, and emotional demands are all fundamental in making a diagnosis. In addition to palpation and stress testing, the physical examination includes an assessment of an athlete's gait, leg length, patellar tracking, and overall limb alignment.

Treatments are primarily directed at changing faulty biomechanics via alterations in running style, a transfer to appropriate running surfaces, and modification of shoewear. Malalignment is treated with corrective orthotics and active rest, with lessened mileage. Stretching exercises—along with strengthening, agility, flexibility, and coordination drills—are reinforced after measures have been taken to correct alignment and quiet the inflammatory process. Rest, non–weight-bearing status, elevation, cryotherapy, compression, mobilization, nonsteroidal antiinflammatory medicines, and heat after 24 to 48 hours all contribute to increase the extensibility of collagen and decrease joint stiffness. Exercises are prescribed early, increasing the load to the limbs within the constraints of pain tolerance. Low-impact activities with minimized gravitational components include pool walking, cross-country skiing, NordicTrack, swimming, and biking. These offer excellent conditioning potentials while minimizing joint reactive forces. Surgery is reserved for those athletes who fail to respond to conservative measures and activity modification. Occasionally excision of scar and degenerated tissue secondary to delayed healing in cases of tendinosis is warranted.

## CONCLUSION

The majority of the injuries discussed in this chapter share similar criteria for evaluation to determine the correct timing for an athlete's return to sport. Compressive dressings, cryotherapy, topical analgesics, and functional bracing can all be used in an effort to accelerate an athlete's resumption of activity. Trial of functional maneuvers can be used to demonstrate an individual's agility and strength and to best elucidate his or her deficits in these areas. Administration of medicines, and particularly the injection of anesthetics and corticosteroids, must be judiciously undertaken. Imprudently or arbitrarily dispensing sensory altering substances can predispose an individual to serious injury for which the medical professional is liable. The medical team treating and ensuring the athlete's physical well-being is well served by erring on the side of being conservative. We cannot rely on the coaches, parents, teammates, and even the athletes themselves to act prudently while tempers and emotions run high in the midst of competition.

## References

1. Andrish JT: The leg. In DeLee JC, Drez D, editors: *Orthopedic and sports medicine principles and practice*, Philadelphia, 1994, WB Saunders.
2. Baxter DE: Functional nerve disorders in the athlete's foot, ankle and leg, *Instr Course Lect* 42:185-194, 1993.
3. Brostrum C: Sprained ankle I: anatomic lesions in recent sprains, *Acta Chir Scand* 128:483-495, 1964.
4. Dupont M, Beliveau P, Theriault G: The efficacy of antiinflammatory medicine in the treatment of the acutely sprained ankle, *Am J Sports Med* 15:41-45, 1987.
5. Eisele SA, Sammarco GJ: Chronic exertional compartment syndrome, *Instr Course Lect* 42:213-217, 1993.
6. Gariffin H, Tropp H, Odenrick P: Effective ankle disc training on postural control in patients with functional instability of the ankle joint, *Int J Sports Med* 9:144, 1988.
7. Hocult JE et al: Cryotherapy in ankle sprains, *Am J Sports Med* 10:316-319, 1982.
8. Jarvinen M, Lehto M: The effective early mobilization and immobilization in the healing process following muscle injuries, *Sports Med* 15:78-89, 1993.
9. Lutter L: Hindfoot problems, *Instr Course Lect* 42:195-200, 1993.
10. McKenzie DC, Clement DB, Taunton JE: Running shoes, orthotics and injuries, *Sports Med* 2:334-347, 1985.
11. Renstrom PAFH: Mechanism, diagnosis, and treatment of running injuries, *Instr Course Lect* 42:225-236, 1993.
12. Renstrom PAFH, Kannus P: Injuries of the foot and ankle. In DeLee JC, Drez D, editors: *Orthopaedic and sports medicine principles and practice*, Philadelphia, 1994, WB Saunders.
13. Renstrom PAFH et al: Strain in the lateral ligaments of the ankle, *Foot Ankle Int* 9:59-63, 1988.
14. Rorabeck CH, Fowler PJ, Nott L: The results of fasciotomy in the management of chronic exertional compartment syndrome, *Am J Sports Med* 16:224-227, 1988.
15. Rovere GD et al: Retrospective comparison of taping and ankle stabilizers in preventing ankle injury, *Am J Sports Med* 16:228-233, 1988.
16. Stanitski C, McMaster J, Scranton P: On the nature of stress fractures, *Am J Sports Med* 6:391-396, 1978.
17. Walter NE, Wolf MD: Stress fractures in young athletes, *Am J Sports Med* 5:165-170, 1977.
18. Woo SLY et al: Treatment of the medial collateral ligament injury, II: Structure and function of canine knees in response to different treatment regimens, *Am J Sports Med* 15:22-29, 1987.

# Chapter 15

# Foot injuries

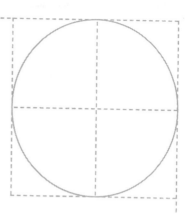

Kenneth W. Bramlett
Ronald G. Derr

Injuries to the foot commonly occur in sports because of the necessity for rapid acceleration, mobility, and change of direction. Among the most common foot injuries in general athletic participation are turf toe, toenail injury, tendon injuries, stress fractures, acute traumatic fractures, articular subluxations and dislocations, and blisters. The definition, mechanism of injury, diagnostic criteria, common treatment, and considerations for return to activity and sports participation for each of these particular injuries of the foot are discussed. The treatment suggested for each injury is especially important during the early stages of the injury (i.e., the first 2 weeks). Early diagnosis, treatment, and rehabilitation will enable the player to return quickly to activity and sports participation.

## TURF TOE

Turf toe injury derives its name from AstroTurf or other artificial playing surfaces.[3,15] This injury is essentially a sprain of the capsuloligamentous structures that stabilize the metatarsophalangeal (MTP) joint of the great toe[3,4,6,18]; it is most commonly encountered in football, baseball, and soccer.[4,5,19] Factors contributing to turf toe injury are lightweight, very flexible shoes commonly worn while playing on artificial surfaces that are hard.[4,5,18] Although this is not considered to be a serious injury, it can become chronically disabling if not treated early and correctly.[3] At the University of Arkansas, turf toe injuries resulted in more decreased player participation time than ankle sprains.[5]

### Mechanism of injury

The three common mechanisms of turf toe injury are hyperextension, hyperflexion, and valgus stress of the MTP joint. Of these, hyperextension is the most common mechanism. This occurs when a player is in the prone position, with the forefoot planted and the heel raised (Fig. 15-1,

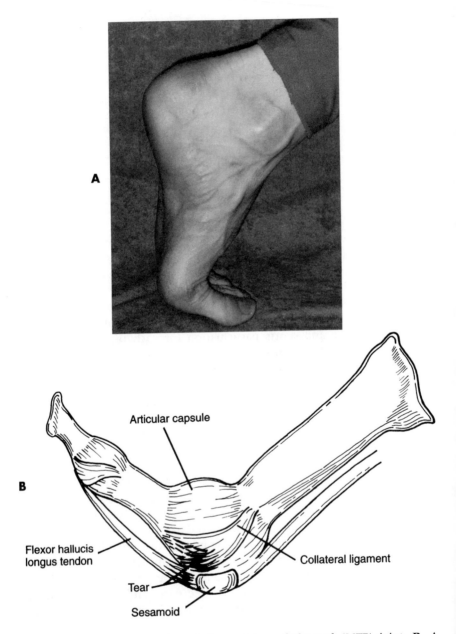

**Fig. 15-1. A,** Hyperextension of the metatarsophalangeal (MTP) joint. **B,** A hyperextension injury of the MTP joint.

*A and B*).[3,5,6,18] As another player falls onto the back of the athlete's leg, the MTP joint is forced past the physiologic limit of extension (approximately 50 degrees).[3,4] This stretches the thick, plantar ligamentous plate that connects the proximal phalanx and metatarsal—causing the weaker proximal metatarsal insertion to tear loose.[3] Flexible shoes commonly worn by players on artificial turf can offer little resistance to MTP hyperextension. In one study, this mechanism accounted for 85% of the turf toe injuries.[18]

The second type of injury mechanism is hyperflexion. This injury occurs when a player is tackled from behind, and the knee is driven forward. In this position, the player's foot is plantarflexed; a second tackler strikes from the front, and the ball carrier is bent back, resulting in hyperflexion of the knee and toe.[5]

The third type of injury mechanism is valgus stress. It most often occurs to offensive linemen during acceleration from their stance into a block or sled formation.[5] Varus stresses can also occur but are infrequent.

**Diagnosis**

Since a turf toe injury is a soft tissue injury, it is diagnosed clinically and is not as evident on radiographs. Radiographs may aid in excluding the possibility of fractures[3-6]—especially fractures of the sesamoid bones beneath the first MTP joint, or small avulsion fractures.

Pain is the most critical and evident symptom of a turf toe injury.[3] With a mild hyperextension injury, the pain is often focal and plantar, whereas with a more severe injury, the pain is usually more diffuse and dorsal.[4] Pain is reproduced with passive range of motion of the first MTP joint in the direction of the injury mechanism. Swelling, ecchymosis, and limited range of motion may result with increasing severity of injury.[4] Clanton and colleagues[4] classified these turf toe injuries into grade I (mild), grade II (moderate), and grade III (severe) injuries. These correspond to a stretch, partial tear, or complete tear of the capsuloligamentous structure (Fig. 15-1, *B*).[15]

**Treatment**

The treatment regimen should include restriction of MTP joint motion, ice, compression, and elevation (RICE).[4,5,6,19] Motion restriction can be accomplished in several ways. A firm, custom-made orthotic can be inserted in the shoe—causing a decrease of MTP joint extension by 25 to 30 degrees. This change will not noticeably affect player mobility.[4] Taping the injury as described by Cooper[5] should be done (in addition to the use of orthotics) but should not be used on swollen toes. A change in the footwear to a less flexible shoe, such as a soccer shoe or a standard seven-cleated football shoe (if playing on natural grass), may prove to be more helpful.

To limit swelling, immediate attention should be given to applyng ice and a compression dressing, and to elevating the foot. Joint mobilization should also be maintained. Injecting the injured area with a local anesthetic and/or a steroid to mask the pain and to allow continued participation is not recommended.[4,5] This approach can worsen the severity of the injury and may result in a possible chronic disability.[4] A nonsteroidal antiinflammatory medication may be used. After the acute injury period, ultrasound, contrast baths, and paraffin can be used.[5]

The player should undergo gradual rehabilitation as tolerated. Shoe modifications and taping may allow for an earlier return to sports participation, but great caution must be observed. Light athletic shoes, such as basketball shoes, worn for football or other similar sports do not support the foot relative to the biomechanical demands and thus should be strongly discouraged.

**Return-to-play criteria**

The time missed from practice or games will depend on the severity of the turf toe injury. A player with a grade I sprain may be able to continue to participate with taping or an orthotic. On the other hand, a player with a grade III sprain may be unable to participate for several weeks. The player needs to undergo gradual rehabilitation with progressively increasing activity.[5] Rehabilitation may start with walking and progress through jogging; running straight ahead; accelerating from a stance; and, finally, cutting. The athlete should continue with each step of activity until discomfort is minimal to nonexistent. Should persistent pain recur, the player should decrease his or her activity to a level that is comfortably tolerable. It is important to maintain an open line of communication with the player about his or her ability to continue to play.

## TOENAIL INJURIES

Toenail injuries can result from various conditions in the athletic environment—such as intensity of play, change-of-direction requirements, and footwear.[9,14,20] There are several types of toenail injuries, including subungual hematomas and ingrown toenails with secondary infections of the surrounding soft tissues.

### SUBUNGUAL HEMATOMA

**Definition**

A subungual hematoma is a collection of extravasated blood beneath the nail plate that is often under pressure.

### Mechanism of injury

Acute trauma, such as a crushing injury or repetitive shear forces to the nail, results in a painful subungual hematoma.[20] The latter mechanism is most commonly seen among athletes involved in contact sports or sports requiring rapid pivoting, and among athletes who run in inadequate footwear. The hematoma will usually appear acutely, but if injury occurs under the proximal nail fold, it may not be evident for 2 to 3 days.[14]

### Diagnosis

Accurate diagnosis necessitates identifying the cause of the injury. Acute crushing types of injuries may involve a distal phalanx fracture or nail bed laceration. A subungual hematoma that develops slowly over weeks to months may be due to a malignant melanoma and must be assessed by a physician.[20] An underlying bony anomaly may be present if there are recurrent problems. X-rays will aid in the diagnosis of a fracture or bony anomaly. When the entire nail surface is involved, it may be necessary to remove the nail plate to evaluate the nail bed for a possible laceration.[20]

### Treatment

Pain can be reduced initially by evacuating the fluid beneath the nail. This is done by making a small hole in the nail plate over the area of the hematoma. This is most easily performed with a heated paper clip, a battery-operated cautery unit, or an 18-gauge needle spun between the fingers.[20] The treatment may be made more comfortable with digital block anesthesia.

If a fracture of the distal phalanx is involved, then the digit will have to be immobilized with a splint or by buddy taping. However, if the fracture is displaced, pinning may be necessary.

As mentioned earlier, a hematoma involving the entire nail surface may have to be removed to repair a laceration of the nail bed. When a melanoma is suspected, a biopsy of the nail bed is necessary.

### Return-to-play criteria

The primary criterion for return to activity is the level of pain that can be tolerated. Participation can resume as tolerated with adequate protection and mobility of the injured area.

## INFECTED INGROWN TOENAIL

### Definition

An infected ingrown toenail refers to the repeated trauma and irritation caused by a nail to the paronychial soft tissue, resulting in secondary infection and inflammation.

### Mechanism of injury

An infected ingrown toenail is caused by a curling or short-edge nail pressing into the paronychial fold. Recurrent abrasion and pressure create soft tissue penetration similar to that caused by a foreign body, and secondary cellulitis may result.

**Diagnosis**

The diagnosis of an infected ingrown toenail is clinical, and x-rays are not necessary. This condition usually occurs in the nail of the great toe. The more focally involved area is commonly the lateral edge. Focal tenderness around the nail edge and redness along the nail fold are observed.

**Treatment**

Prevention is the best treatment for an infected ingrown toenail. Instruction on nail trimming and choosing comfortable shoes should be provided to the player. Once inflamed and tender, nail irritation can be alleviated by packing cotton beneath the edge of the nail and by paronychial retraction on a repeated basis.

Once infection and extreme pain are present, oral antibiotic treatment and nail edge resection under digital block anesthesia can be useful methods of treatment. For recurrent cases, partial nail resection is a very effective treatment; yet complete nail resection is not advised (Fig. 15-2, A and B).

**Return-to-play criteria**

A player with an ingrown toenail can participate in sports at any time unless the discomfort inhibits necessary performance levels.

# TENDON INJURIES

## POSTERIOR TIBIAL TENDINITIS

### Definition

Posterior tibial tendinitis is often seen as an overuse injury in sports that necessitate running, jumping, or strong push-off actions.[1,8] Tenosynovitis is probably a more accurate term because the inflammation is confined to the synovial sheath around the tendon, and not the tendon itself. Posterior tibial tendinitis is much more common than posterior tibial tendon rupture, which is rarely seen among the athletic population.[8] However, tendon rupture and attritional tears may be frequently observed with an aging population who continue athletic activity into their later years.

### Diagnosis

A younger player with posterior tibial tendinitis complains of pain along the posterior aspect of the medial malleolus that radiates into the medial lower leg. Such a player usually has a history of stepping into a hole, twisting the ankle, or incurring pain along the medial calf and arch with push-off and acceleration. The clinical exam by palpation reveals

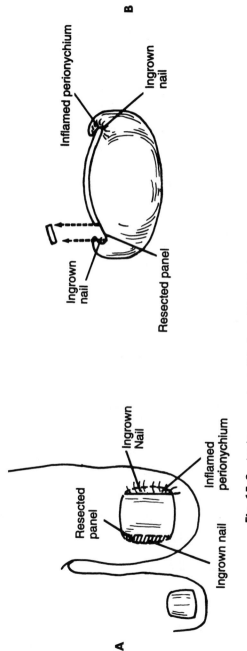
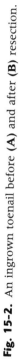

**Fig. 15-2.** An ingrown toenail before (**A**) and after (**B**) resection.

tenderness along the course of the tendon, often originating from the navicular insertion. The integrity of the tendon can best be confirmed by having the player perform a series of unilateral toe raises. Relative weakness may be noted when comparing pain on the injured side with the opposite side.[8] Patients with severe cases may even complain of calf pain in the medial gastrocnemius muscle, and occasionally radiation of pain into the popliteal region may be noted. Thrombophlebitis, fracture, periostitis, and rupture of the posterior tibial tendon must be considered in the differential diagnosis.

When a rupture of the posterior tibial tendon occurs, players usually experience a "popping" sensation along the medial ankle or foot. Examination shows a collapse in the medial longitudinal arch, and the player is unable to perform unilateral toe raises. If the tendon has been ruptured completely, full double-leg and single-leg weight bearing is intolerable. Another useful diagnostic tool is to view the standing player from behind. From this viewing position it will appear that the player has more toes lateral to the heel on the injured side, (i.e., the "too many toes" sign).[8] X-rays do not add significantly to the diagnosis but should be performed to rule out bone pathology.

**Treatment**

Tendinitis can be treated like any inflammatory condition—with ice, rest (if necessary), and possibly a nonsteroidal antiinflammatory medication. A custom-made shoe insert or an orthotic that incorporates a good arch support can aid in reducing any excess strain on the tendon resulting from early collapse of the midfoot arch. This is the most effective preventive and acute postinjury treatment for both tendinitis and a partial tear. Most commonly, pes cavus feet or feet with transitioning midfoot collapse have an overworked posterior tibial tendon that results in tendinitis. Adequate orthotic midfoot support can provide even weight distribution to the plantar sole and rest to the tendon unit to relieve this condition. Once posterior tibial tendinitis is diagnosed, prevention of progressive symptoms is the best treatment.

To help prevent recurrence, it is important to strengthen and stretch the posterior tibial muscle through focal physical therapy. For acute cases, in which players have severe pain or chronic symptoms, a short-leg walking cast with a well-molded arch can be advantageous. This period of immobilization should be followed with a custom dynamic insert (CDI)–molded orthotic to support compromised hindfoot and midfoot mechanics.

Posterior tibial tendon rupture can be treated with conservative measures such as casting, physical therapy, CDI orthotics, and a gradual return to play (Fig. 15-3, *A* and *B*). If these measures are not effective, surgery may be necessary. Once surgical repair is performed, gradual

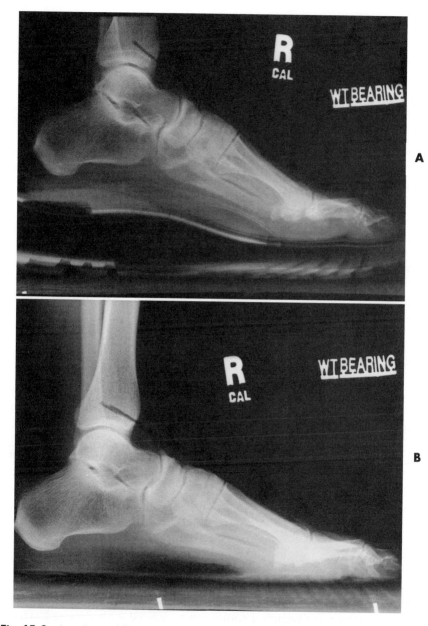

**Fig. 15-3.** A patient with posterior tibial tendinitis. **A,** The left shoe and orthotic are on, thereby supporting the midfoot. **B,** The left shoe is off, picturing collapse of the arch when a custom dynamic insert (CDI) is not used.

rehabilitation is necessary—along with full-time orthotic support and appropriate shoewear for life.

**Return-to-play criteria**

As soon as the player has undergone a complete foot and ankle evaluation, return to activity may be possible. However, long-term precautions that include wearing appropriate shoes, using orthotics, and avoiding activity overload should be considered to prevent recurrence or worsening of tendinitis symptoms.

## STRESS FRACTURES

### Definition

A stress fracture is an overuse injury to a bone that results when nonviolent stress is applied in a cyclic, repetitive, subthreshold manner. This fracture may lead to a partial or complete fracture.[8,13] Stress fractures can occur in any bone of the foot, with certain bones (i.e., the metatarsals) more prone than others. The terms "stress lesion" and "stress reaction" refer to the earliest stress remodeling phase of bone before fracture occurs.[13] X-rays of these lesions are not positive initially. However, stress fractures are radiographically positive.

### Mechanism of injury

A stress fracture usually results from an acute change in a training routine, such as a rapid increase in training mileage or sessions. The fracture may result from any weight-bearing activity that stresses the bone beyond its ability to recover. This can occur in a foot with normal, as well as abnormal, biomechanics. The foot that possesses altered biomechanics commonly develops symptoms at an earlier stage. Certain types of abnormalities may lead to their own particular stress fracture patterns. Cavus feet, which are inclined to be more rigid, generally experience metatarsal shaft fractures. Less rigid, pronated feet are more likely to suffer stress fractures of the navicula, talus, and tibia.[1] Certain activities can also produce a typical stress fracture pattern. Marching frequently leads to metatarsal shaft injuries, whereas hurtling, because of the repetitive landing on a plantarflexed foot, more often causes stress fractures of the tarsal navicula (Fig. 15-4, *A* and *B*).

### Diagnosis

Pain is the most common complaint associated with a stress fracture. The initial pain of a stress fracture may be an ache or soreness of gradual onset, but it is always activity-related. Swelling may accompany this pain. With a short period of rest, the pain may subside until the player reaches the threshold of stress for reinjuring the bone. A player with a high tolerance for pain may be able to continue to participate despite the injury;

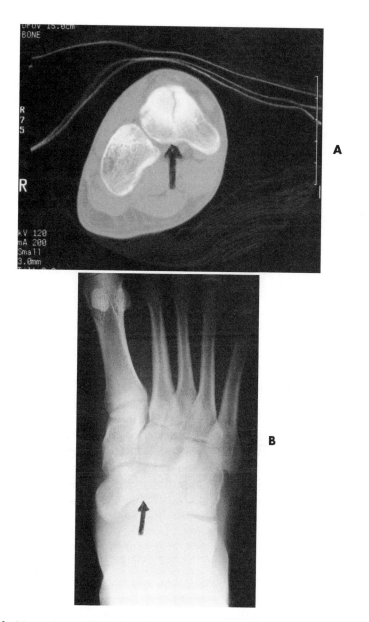

**Fig. 15–4.** Magnetic resonance imaging (MRI) **(A)** and an x-ray **(B)** of the same navicular stress fracture.

however, the activity should be discontinued to prevent any further damage, and medical advice should be sought.

Examination frequently demonstrates focal pain with palpation over the affected bone. Patients can often communicate the area and severity of pain quite accurately. Stressing a long bone in the foot over a fulcrum at the area of suspected injury will increase the pain response. On palpating the calcaneus, pain is found to be present on the sides of the bone and not on the plantar aspect. Vibration of the involved bone with a tuning fork may also be valuable since pain may be generated at the fracture site.

Plain radiographs initially may not reveal a stress fracture for 3 to 4 weeks. If bone changes cannot be identified on a plain x-ray, other imaging tests can be used if there is doubt. A triple phase bone scan (TPBS) is the imaging test of choice because it assists in evaluating stress injuries. In the earliest (stress remodeling) and latest (healing) phases of a stress fracture, only the delayed phase will be positive. During the hyperemic period of the acute stress fracture, all three phases will be positive. TPBS is very effective when combined with a patient history, a thorough examination, and a plain x-ray.[13] In a highly suspicious injury, if a TPBS is negative, technical factors must be considered as the cause. Computer subtraction methods and/or single photon emission computed tomography (SPECT) scans may also be helpful. If necessary, a 24-hour delayed image should be obtained, before considering the scan negative.[13] Magnetic resonance imaging (MRI) may be used as a diagnostic tool but usually is not necessary.

**Early treatment**

As soon as a stress fracture is suspected, treatment should begin immediately to avoid any difficulty that could cause delays with definitive diagnosis. Early treatment consists of decreased activity or complete rest (i.e., casting). The necessity for initial casting or even surgical fixation depends on the stability of the fracture. Fractures considered unstable or "at risk" include those of the navicular, proximal fifth metatarsal, sesamoid, and all intraarticular fractures.[8] These fractures have a higher risk of displacement, delayed or nonunion healing of the fracture, complete fracture, or permanent morbidity. Once stability is assured, either with or without surgery, an individualized rehabilitation program can be implemented.

Stable fractures, such as metatarsal fractures, necessitate monitoring as the rehabilitation program continues and the healing progresses. Os calcis stress fractures are very stable but can necessitate an extended period of time to become asymptomatic. Activity modification accompanied by stretching and strengthening exercises of the intrinsics and the extrinsics of the foot should begin early in rehabilitation. Mechanical support, such as orthotics or firm-soled shoes, can be used. Running can be allowed in some cases, at a level at which symptoms of stress fracture do not reappear. Cycling and swimming enable aerobic training to continue without discomfort.

**Proximal fifth metatarsal stress fracture.** Once identified, proximal fifth metatarsal fractures in athletes must be treated attentively using open or closed methods. Factors to be considered for the treatment are the nature of the injury and the particular sport under consideration.

For a first-time, nondisplaced fracture of the proximal fifth metatarsal, casting may be effective. Closed treatment in a cast may require 4 to 8 weeks to obtain a nonpainful level of walking in the cast. Monitoring for any reinjury must be done as rehabilitation and conditioning resume. If pain or delayed union persists following closed treatment, then open treatment may be considered.

For athletes participating in running, contact, or jumping sports, open techniques are our preferred choice for proximal fifth metatarsal fractures that are caused by stress and repetitive use. Open fixation allows immediate fixation for the displaced and nondisplaced injuries, and it provides for an earlier return to conditioning activities such as cycling and swimming. Open intramedullary fixation with a 4-mm cancellous screw shortens the inactive period of the recovery phase and allows for an earlier and more confident return to full athletic participation.

Following open intramedullary fixation of a proximal fifth metatarsal fracture, 2 to 4 weeks of casting may be used to allow progressive weight bearing and comfort. Once pain is minimal, casting is discontinued; cycling and swimming may then begin. As full range of motion and weight bearing become possible during the 4- to 8-week recovery process—and corresponding to clinical and radiographic assessment—progressive running on a flat surface may begin with cutting and jumping drills.

Once each phase of recovery has been completed, full return to play is possible (usually occurring during the 6- to 10-week postoperative interval). Note that recovery with any fracture is dependent on the individual, the nature of the fracture, and the treatment technique variables. The benefit of secure open fixation is a decreased risk of delayed union or recurrence of proximal fifth metatarsal fractures.

**Navicular stress fracture.** Navicular stress fractures may occur in athletes involved in repetitive running sports such as cross-country or hurdling.[12] The repetitive impact of the forefoot onto a flat or an irregular surface creates focal stresses that are transmitted through the midfoot navicular region as the foot adjusts for impact, stance, and push-off during the running cycle.

During the initial period, clinically the patient with a midfoot stress fracture may experience vague (i.e., nonfocal) pain, which is located in the midfoot medially and has symptoms radiating into the forefoot along the first and the second metatarsal.[22] A careful clinical history and physical exam combined with a standard foot x-ray and a supplemental TPBS may be very helpful in the diagnostic process. Yet often radiographic findings may be delayed 1 to 2 months following the onset of midfoot pain.[23]

The pain of a navicular fracture may be made worse by requesting the patient to stand on the toes and extend downward pressure onto the metatarsal heads to exacerbate the symptoms[12]; this may be helpful in assessing suspected navicular injuries.

Stress fractures of the navicular may be radiographically confused with bipartite navicular development; yet, when present, they are commonly found in the central third region of the bone in a sagittal orientation.[22]

Once diagnosed, our preferred treatment is dependent on the stage of the injury to the navicular. Early diagnosis of a navicular stress fracture is commonly associated with vague pain along the talonavicular joint. Bone scans may be positive, yet computed tomography (CT) scans and MRIs may show early sclerotic changes in the subchondral navicular zone and the extent of the fracture line progression. If radiographs reveal minimal sclerotic changes in the subchondral region of the proximal navicular surface—and if limited fracture line penetrations exist—then immobilization for 3 months, with nonimpact conditioning and observation for progressive improvement of symptoms, is the treatment option.[22] Repeat CT or MRI assessment may be performed in 3 months and clinically correlated.

Late diagnosis of a navicular stress fracture is associated with more focal and more intense pain at the midfoot talonavicular articulation. A positive bone scan, as well as a CT scan or MRI revealing a linear fracture line of the navicular and sclerotic bone changes along the fracture line, is usually reported. At this stage, it is our preference to intervene in the progression of the navicular fracture process. Radiographs reveal sclerosis, a linear fracture line, and the development of displacement. Open debridement of the sclerotic navicular margins and supplementation with autogenous interbody navicular bone graft and transfracture fixation is the preferred method.

After autogenous grafting and fixation of the navicular fracture, conservative management in a cast is provided for 8 to12 weeks. During the first 8 weeks, only touch-down weight bearing (TDWB) is allowed. Once initial immobilization is completely progressive, activities allowing force control across the navicular may be started. Noncontact conditioning programs—including cycling, swimming, and progressive walking—may be used during the recovery period. Full return to play may occur at the 6- to 9-month postoperation interval if clinical and radiographic findings are complementary.

## Return-to-play criteria

The earlier a stress fracture is diagnosed and appropriate treatment initiated, the sooner the player will be able to return to play. A stable stress fracture may only limit participation for a few weeks until symptoms decrease or disappear. An unstable injury that necessitates casting or surgery may take 8 to 12 weeks to heal, with an additional period of time to regain adequate conditioning.

Specifically, stress fractures of the proximal fifth metatarsal and stress fractures of the navicular are problem fractures for competitive athletes. Diffuse pain initially may develop, yet repetitive activities may exacerbate the focal discomfort. Because of the insidious onset of these fractures, they may be initially overlooked.

Fractures of the proximal fifth metatarsal cause posterolateral foot pain radiating along the peroneal tendons and may be associated with a "pop" or focal strain during performance. The best initial treatment is usually immobilization of the lower extremity, preferably in a cast; yet if displacement exists and pain is not relieved by initial casting, open fixation with a longitudinally placed intramedullary screw may be curative. Plain x-rays may initially be diagnostic, yet bone scans may assist in stress fracture diagnosis when standard radiographs are inconclusive.

The navicular stress fracture develops in athletes who transmit excessive force through the midfoot (i.e., hurdlers). Insidious pain in the midfoot may be noted, which is worsened by the frequency of activity and the level of impact applied to the foot. Bone scans may assist in the diagnosis of navicular stress fractures since plain films commonly do not reveal these fractures in the early stages. CT scans are specifically diagnostic and may include both the depth and direction of the fracture, thereby assisting in the planning of fixation. CT scans may reveal sclerotic margins that may develop along the fracture line of chronic navicular stress fractures.

Once navicular fractures are diagnosed, open treatment is commonly necessary. Postoperative casting is implemented and TDWB is allowed, usually for 6 weeks, with progressive weight bearing during the second 6 weeks. Conditioning exercises of both the upper and lower body may continue during the 3-month recovery phase. Return to competition is generally not allowed until symptoms abate and radiographs support the clinical assessment.

# FRACTURES

## Definition

Besides fatigue or stress fractures (discussed earlier), other fractures include all acute injuries to the bone that lead to a complete disruption of the bone cortex. These include nondisplaced fractures, displaced fractures, and avulsion fractures. Fracture displacement refers to the positional relationship of the individual fracture fragments to each other. Nondisplaced fractures have fractured surfaces that are in complete apposition to each other and have a normal alignment in all planes. Displaced fractures have partial or complete loss of apposition and/or alignment of their individual fracture fragments. Avulsion fractures occur in the region of the bone where the ligament or tendon attachment is under acute, excessive tension that causes the bone to break. In other words, bone failure occurs before connective tissue failure (Fig. 15-5). Fractures generally are classified as open or closed, depending on whether there is direct communication with the outside environment through a break in the skin at or near the fracture site.

### Mechanism of injury

Unlike stress fractures—which result from a cyclic, repetitive, subthreshold loading of the bone—acute traumatic fractures are caused by one isolated event. Phalangeal fracture is the most common acute forefoot fracture and occurs most frequently when the foot is struck by a dropped object. The remaining bones of the foot are usually fractured when an object strikes the foot of the player or the player lands incorrectly. An avulsion fracture occurs when a joint is extended beyond its maximum limit of motion, and bone failure occurs before the ligament failure. A similar situation occurs with a tendinous avulsion, which results when a sudden maximal force is applied to the tendon attachment. A common avulsion fracture in the foot occurs to the peroneus brevis tendon on the fifth metatarsal base. This results when the peroneus brevis contracts suddenly to prevent foot inversion (e.g., when a player steps in a hole or lands on the lateral aspect of the foot when jumping) (Fig. 15-5).[17]

### Diagnosis

Pain, swelling, tenderness, ecchymosis, crepitance, and deformity are common diagnostic symptoms of fracture. Swelling and ecchymosis may manifest immediately, but they may also take 12 to 24 hours to appear. An antalgic gait may be present and will hinder the performance of the injured athlete. Often a sprain and a fracture will be difficult to differentiate on-site initially, and definitive diagnosis will require a plain x-ray. It is very important initially that the examiner determine whether an open or closed fracture has occurred. When an acute traumatic fracture occurs, the neurovascular integrity of the affected extremity must be documented. All open fractures must receive immediate medical treatment.

### Treatment

Fractures of the foot will usually require some form of immobilization. Immobilization can be external, internal, or a combination of both forms.

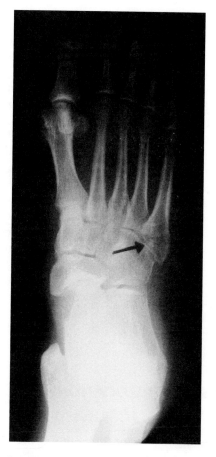

**Fig. 15-5.** A radiograph showing a fifth metatarsal avulsion.

An external form of immobilization may be a cast, splint, or cast boot; internal immobilization can be accomplished using pins or screws. If significant displacement is present, reduction under local or general anesthesia will be necessary before immobilization. After 3 to 4 weeks of immobilization, many nondisplaced fractures will have healed adequately enough to allow a gradual return to activity. Complete fracture healing may not take place for several more weeks. There is no way to expedite the healing process; however, inadequate treatment can significantly delay healing.

Phalangeal fractures are treated with reduction, if necessary, under digital block anesthesia. This is followed by buddy taping the fractured toe to the normal neighboring toe, which acts as a splint. While taping toes, it is important to pay attention to swelling in order to avoid compromising blood flow. Fractures of the fifth metatarsal tuberosity can be treated with a short-leg walking cast or with crutches and a wooden-soled shoe. Sesamoid fractures should be treated initially with a short-leg walking cast to control pain. Acute fractures of the remaining bones of the foot probably will necessitate splinting initially until swelling and pain have decreased. This is followed by short-leg casting until the fracture heals. Casts are preferred initially for most foot fractures to stabilize the fracture, control pain and swelling, and enhance patient mobilization with less dependence on crutches.

**Return-to-play criteria**

Complete fractures of the bone of the foot, unlike fractures of the hand, are difficult to protect sufficiently to allow continued athletic participation without significantly restricting mobility and performance. Toe fractures are an exception to this fact, especially fractures of the lesser toes. Athletes with midfoot fractures and avulsions will usually be restricted from participation until adequate healing has taken place. However, aerobic and general conditioning can continue in a non–weight-bearing manner. A firm-soled shoe or insert may be helpful on return to activity to dissipate forces away from the injury area. Players should be instructed about their care by the orthopedic surgeon or team athletic trainer.

## SUBLUXATIONS AND DISLOCATIONS

**Definition**

Subluxations and dislocations of the joints of the foot occur in sports. With these injuries, if spontaneous reduction has not occurred, the resulting deformity makes the diagnosis quite evident. When spontaneous reduction has occurred, a description of the mechanism of injury should lead to a "suspicion" of the injury. To clarify the two types of injury, a subluxation is an incomplete dislocation of a joint with partial joint congruity remaining, whereas a dislocation indicates a complete loss of joint congruity.[21] The direction of subluxation or dislocation is named by the position of the distal segment in relation to the proximal segment.[8]

**Mechanism of injury**

The injury mechanisms vary depending on the joint of the foot that is involved. Involvement of the toe joints (i.e., interphalangeal and metatarsophalangeal) is usually due to a violent hyperextension mechanism or to the dropping of a heavy object onto the toes.

Injuries to Lisfranc's joint (i.e., the tarsometatarsal joint in the midfoot arch) occur by either direct or indirect mechanisms. In sports, crushing injury to the foot occurs when there is direct impact to the tarsometatarsal area. On the other hand, the indirect mechanism that is the more common of the two occurs when the foot is in the forced plantarflexion position with a possibility of combined midfoot rotation. This can occur in four possible ways: longitudinal compression (football), falling backward with the forefoot entrapped (horseback riding, wind surfing), falling onto the point of the toes (ballet, dance), and forced forefoot abduction.[8] The diagnosis of a ligament injury to the foot with an associated subluxation of a congruous articulation (i.e., Lisfranc's injury) is difficult and must be considered during the examination.

A subtalar dislocation is referred to as "basketball foot" because of the nature of its occurrence and because it is not a common injury.[12] It occurs when a basketball player, following a rebound or jump shot, lands on the plantarflexed foot—forcing it into supination and causing subtalar dislocation.[7] Only a small amount of force is necessary for this injury to occur.[7] This causes a dislocation most commonly in the medial direction to the talocalcaneal and talonavicular joints.[7,8]

**Diagnosis**

Dislocations and subluxations are not usually difficult to diagnose because of the presence of deformity. However, it may be difficult to determine exactly which joint is involved until plain x-rays are obtained since there is immediate swelling in the injured area. It is important to examine the foot carefully because fractures are very commonly associated with dislocation and subluxation.[8] Often, small avulsion fractures are present because of the ligamentous attachments surrounding the joints. Stress x-rays may be necessary to completely expose the injury (if spontaneous reduction occurs following a suspected dislocation) in conjunction with pain in the joint area and difficulty in weight bearing. Especially with Lisfranc's injuries, bony anatomic relationships must be confirmed with x-rays. The medial border of the fourth metatarsal should be in alignment with the medial border of the cuboid on the oblique x-ray. Additionally, the intermetatarsal separation between the third and fourth metatarsal bases should be continuous with the spacing between the lateral cuneiform and cuboid bones. Likewise, the intermetatarsal separation between the second and third metatarsal bases should correspond with the middle and lateral cuneiform bones. On the anteroposterior view, the medial border of the second metatarsal should be aligned with the medial border of the middle cuneiform bone. Additionally, there should be no increased diastasis between the first and second metatarsal bases as compared with the opposite, normal foot (Fig. 15-6, *A*).[7]

With any fracture or dislocation, the neurovascular status of the foot should be evaluated at the time of injury and periodically until reduction is performed. This is necessary to avoid an extended period of vascular compromise to the foot and to the skin tented over any

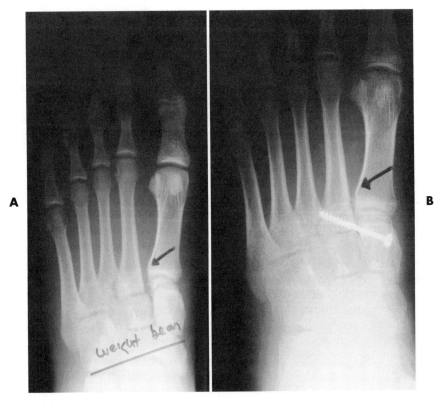

**Fig. 15-6. A,** A weight-bearing anteroposterior x-ray of a foot—revealing a Lisfranc's injury with separation of the first and second metatarsal bases. **B,** A follow-up anteroposterior x-ray of the same foot after open fixation.

bony prominences.[7,8] Neurovascular evaluation is performed by palpating pedal pulses and by visually checking the capillary refill of the toes and the color of the skin. If indicated, urgent reduction may be necessary.

**Treatment**

Immediate treatment on the field should include neurovascular checks, an evaluation for open injury, and splinting to stabilize the injury in the position in which it is found. Immediate transport to a medical facility should be arranged for the following reasons: (1) the sooner the joint is reduced, the more comfortable the player will be; (2) reduction is often easier to perform before soft tissue spasm and significant swelling occur; (3) any areas affected by ischemia of the skin, noted by blanching—especially when tented over a bony prominence—must be relieved of the pressure as soon as possible to avoid skin necrosis.

If obvious acute malposition of the hindfoot or midfoot occurs and medical intervention is delayed with uncertainty, it is advisable to reduce the foot acutely. By applying slow, progressively increasing, longitudinal traction to the foot, the severity of the pain and prolonged vascular compromise caused by a hindfoot or midfoot dislocation can be greatly reduced. With relocation, significant pain will be reduced (thereby avoiding potential shock) and bone or joint disruption is seldom made worse.[8]

Once x-rays are obtained, a closed reduction maneuver can be performed in the hospital or clinic setting under the comfort of a local, regional, or general anesthetic. If the injury is open or if closed reduction is unsuccessful, then irrigation, debridement, or open reduction with internal fixation may be necessary (Fig. 15-6, *A* and *B*).

Following a subluxation-dislocation injury to the foot, early range of motion is strongly encouraged in most cases. This may begin following a 3- to 4-week period of immobilization in a short-leg cast, with weight bearing allowed as tolerated by the patient.[8] With lesser toe interphalangeal dislocations, closed reduction and buddy taping will usually be adequate treatment, with no restrictions on weight bearing. Depending on the involvement of the sesamoids, dislocations of the digital metatarsophalangeal may necessitate open reduction. This is followed by short-leg casting or possibly the use of a wooden-soled shoe for 3 to 4 weeks.

Aggressive treatment of a Lisfranc's disruption injury is encouraged for long-term results. This usually means percutaneous pinning or open anatomic reduction with internal fixation (Fig. 15-6, *B*).[7]

### Return-to-play criteria

Because of the weight-bearing nature of the foot, dislocation of joints other than the toes may keep a player inactive for several weeks or months and may even end a career. Therefore it is important that these injuries be evaluated and treated by an orthopedic surgeon who will closely monitor the injury. With toe injuries, full, painless range of motion is needed for the player to return to play. With subtalar dislocations, there is a possibility of avascular necrosis of the talus or early osteoarthritis of the subtalar joint. During the first year postinjury, progress must be closely monitored using periodic bone scans and x-rays to watch for the aforementioned complications. A negative bone scan is preferred before return to athletic activity. Thereafter, periodic negative bone scans will aid in follow-up.[8] With Lisfranc's injuries, players should not be allowed to return to play until they have full, painless range of motion of the injured joint, along with no residual inflammation or signs of early osteoarthritis.[8] A custom-made orthotic with longitudinal and metatarsal arch support should be used to support the foot.

## BLISTERS

### Definition

A blister is a fluid-filled vesicle under the epidermis (subepidermal) or within the epidermis (intradermal).[11,21] The fluid filling the vesicle can be either serum or blood. Blisters most commonly occur on the hands and the feet where the epidermal skin layer is tightly bound to the underlying tissues. In the foot, blisters are usually caused by shearing forces brought on by friction between the skin and another material (i.e., socks, shoes). Blisters are often considered insignificant injuries that cause only temporary discomfort, but they can lead to compromised individual performance.[11] Without proper treatment they can progress to ulceration, cellulitis, local infection, or sepsis.[16]

### Mechanism of injury

Friction blisters, commonly seen on the foot in sports, are caused by shearing forces between the skin and another surface.[2,11,16] The skin reacts by either thickening or blistering in an attempt to protect the deeper tissues from this trauma.

Blister formation follows a two step process. First, shear forces cause tearing of the epidermal skin layers, allowing a cleft to form in the mid to upper malpighian layer. This leaves a roof consisting of the stratum corneum, lucidum, and granulosum.[11,16] Second, the cleft is filled with fluid by the local hemodynamic forces. Skin moisture and temperature are contributing factors—with warm, moist skin blistering easier than skin that is cool, dry, or very wet.[2,11,16]

### Treatment

Prevention with proper shoes, socks, and other preventive products is the primary treatment for friction blisters. Shoes should fit properly and should be sport-specific, if possible, rather than of the "all purpose" or "cross-training" type. Socks that allow air to reach the skin while wicking away moisture are highly recommended.[11] Multiple layers of socks (double or triple) decrease the shear forces significantly.[16] It has been demonstrated that socks made of acrylic cause fewer and smaller blisters than cotton socks in runners.[11] Preventive products include powders (to dry), padded insoles (to cushion), lubricating agents, and skin tougheners. Gradual increase in activity is recommended.[1]

Once a blister forms, treatment should provide comfort, rapid healing, and prevention of infection.[16] This is best accomplished using conservative measures and can be carried out by the player if instructed properly.

Unroofing the blister appears to be an important question during treatment. Literature supports both options of maintaining the roof and unroofing the blister.[2,10,16] The authors tend to be in agreement with the treatment plan as described by Ramsey.[16] Ruptured, tattered blisters should be debrided of loose skin and cleansed with hydrogen peroxide or warm soapy water 2 or 3 times daily until the blister is healed or the peroxide fails to foam. Minimally torn or untorn blisters should remain covered with skin, which will adhere to the base and provide protection and more rapid healing. The untorn blisters should be decompressed with aseptic aspiration or lancing, repeated as necessary the first few days, to allow for adhesion of top to base. If the blister is unroofed, an antibiotic ointment should be applied to the base following each cleansing. Regardless of whether it has a roof or not, the lesion should be bandaged to protect and maintain decompression. Additional padding with felt or foam can be used for further protection if necessary.[2,16]

If signs of infection appear (i.e., red streaks radiating from the blister or the development of a purulent discharge) medical advice should be sought. A short course of intravenous and/or oral antibiotics might be necessary to fight the infection.

**Return-to-play criteria**

Return to play can occur as quickly as the individual player can tolerate. A mild infection that is being treated with oral antibiotics and protected sufficiently should not prevent the player from participating in sports. Prevention of further blistering, as discussed previously, should be pursued aggressively on return to activity.

## References

1. Baxter DE: The foot in running. In Mann RA, Coughlin MJ, editors: *Surgery of the foot and ankle,* ed 6, St Louis, 1993, Mosby–Year Book.
2. Bergfeld WF, Taylor JS: Trauma, sports and the skin, *Am J Ind Med* 8:403-413, 1985.
3. Bowers KD, Martin RB: Turf-toe: a shoe surface related football injury, *Med Sci Sports Exerc* 8:81-83, 1976.
4. Clanton TO, Barnes JE, Eggert A: Injuries to the metatarsophalangeal joints in athletes, *Foot Ankle Int* 7:162-176, 1986.
5. Coker TP, Arnold JA, Weber DL: Traumatic lesions of the metatarsophalangeal joint of the great toe in athletes, *Am J Sports Med* 6:139, 1978.
6. Cooper DL: Turf toe, *Physician Sports Med* 6:139, 1978.
7. DeLee JC: Fractures and dislocations of the foot. In Mann RA, Coughlin MJ, editors: *Surgery of the foot and ankle,* ed 6, St Louis, 1993, Mosby–Year Book.
8. DeLee JC, Drez D Jr: *Orthopedic sports medicine: principles and practice,* Philadelphia, 1994, WB Saunders.
9. Eisele SA: Conditions of the toenails, *Orthop Clin North Am* 25:183-188, 1994.
10. Fletcher SB, Whitehill WR, Wright KE: Medicated compress for blister treatment, *J Athletic Train* 28:81-82, 1993.
11. Herring KM, Richie DH Jr: Friction blisters and sock fiber composition: a double-blind study, *J Am Podiatr Assoc* 80:63-71, 1990.
12. Hunter LY: Stress fractures of the tarsal navicular. In Mann RA, Coughlin MJ, editors: *Surgery of the foot and ankle,* ed 6, St Louis, 1993, Mosby–Year Book.
13. Martire JR: Differentiating stress fracture from periostitis, *Physician Sports Med* 22:71-81, 1994.

14. Mortimer PS, Dawber RP: Trauma to the nail unit including occupational sports injuries, *Dermatol Clin* 3:415-420, 1985.
15. Mullis DL, Miller WE: A disabling sports injury of the great toe, *Foot Ankle Int* 1:22-25, 1980.
16. Ramsey ML: Managing friction blisters of the feet, *Physician Sports Med* 20:117-124, 1992.
17. Rockwood CA Jr, Green DP, Bocholz RW: *Rockwood and Green's fractures in adults,* ed 3, Philadelphia, 1991, JB Lippincott.
18. Rodeo SA, O'Brien S, Warren RF, et al: Turf-toe: an analysis of metatarsophalangeal joint sprains in professional football players, *Am J Sports Med* 18:280-285, 1990.
19. Sammarco GJ: How I manage turf toe, *Physician Sports Med* 16:113-118, 1988.
20. Scioli M: Managing toenail trauma, *Physician Sports Med* 20:107-111, 1992.
21. *Stedman's medical dictionary,* ed 24, Baltimore-London, 1982, Williams & Wilkins.
22. Torg JS, Pavlov H, Cooley LH et al: Stress fractures of the tarsal navicular. In Mann RA, Coughlin MJ, editors: *Surgery of the foot and ankle,* ed 6, St Louis, 1993, Mosby–Year Book.
23. Towne LC, Blazina ME, Cozen LN: Fatigue fracture of the tarsal navicular. In Mann RA, Coughlin MJ, editors: *Surgery of the foot and ankle,* ed 6, St Louis, 1993, Mosby–Year Book.

# Chapter 16

# Shoulder injuries

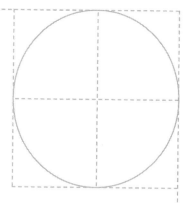

Timothy B. Sutherland

Injuries to the shoulder are common in athletic competition. Appropriate treatment of these injuries necessitates accurate on-field evaluation and diagnosis. Diagnosis is aided by an understanding of the basic anatomy of the shoulder. The shoulder girdle itself consists of the following articulations: the glenohumeral joint; the acromioclavicular joint; the scapulothoracic joint; and the rotator cuff, consisting of the subscapularis, supraspinatus, infraspinatus, and teres minor.

## CLINICAL EVALUATION

Before examination, an accurate history must be obtained. The athlete's complaint must be determined, and the location of the pain noted. The quality, duration, and type of pain should be defined. The athlete should be carefully questioned regarding any neurologic symptoms or pain in the neck. The mechanism of injury should be elucidated. Of particular importance are whether the injury was a contact or noncontact injury and the position of the arm at injury. Careful observation of the field of play can often allow one to observe the injury directly as it occurs. Review of game films or videos can also be helpful in determining the exact time and mechanism of injury.

A complete physical exam allows accurate diagnosis of most common shoulder injuries. When possible, evaluation of the injured athlete should be done on the sideline, off the playing field itself. If the athlete is examined on the field, significant neck, back, or head injuries should be ruled out and the player moved to the sideline for complete evaluation.

Examination of the shoulder begins with removing the player's uniform (shoulder pads and so on) so that both shoulders may be visualized and palpated adequately. The skin should be carefully examined for evidence of abrasions, lacerations, swelling, or ecchymosis. Any abrasions should be appropriately treated at this time. Evidence of skin disruption with an underlying fracture or dislocation constitutes an open (or compound) fracture or dislocation; the injury should be treated as a medical emergency, with immediate transfer of the athlete to a hospital for cleansing and stabilization of the injury. Careful and gentle palpation of the shoulder should then be done to locate the point of maximum tenderness. Any crepitus consistent with an underlying fracture should be noted at this time. Palpation of the neck should always be done to rule out concomitant neck injury. A careful neurovascular examination is then completed. The upper extremity is checked with regard to sensation and compared with the contralateral, uninjured extremity. Motor examination is then done, beginning with the examination of the distal hand and arm and proceeding to the examination of the shoulder.

Active range of motion and strength of the shoulder should be checked in forward flexion, abduction, adduction, external rotation with the arm at the side (0 degrees of abduction), internal rotation with the arm at the side (0 degrees of adduction), and with the empty can test (forward flexion in 30 degrees of horizontal abduction with internal rotation). Each musculotendinous unit can be palpated as active motion is accomplished. Passive range of motion is then evaluated in rotation at 0 degrees of adduction, abduction, and forward flexion. Vascular examination should then be done with palpation of the radial and ulnar pulses at the wrist and observation of the capillary refill. The glenohumeral joint should then be examined for evidence of instability. Anterior and posterior drawer tests of the humeral head in the glenoid should be done with abduction to 90 degrees and external rotation of the arm in the supine position. The acromioclavicular joint should be checked for superior translation (as compared with the contralateral side) and anterior and posterior translation.

## FRACTURES OF THE SHOULDER GIRDLE

Fractures about the shoulder are uncommon in young athletes. They occur most frequently in contact sports secondary to a direct blow. Typical signs of fracture include crepitus over the fractured bone, rapid swelling, and extreme pain.

## CLAVICLE FRACTURES

A clavicle fracture is most common secondary to an indirect force transferred to the clavicle during a hard fall on the outstretched hand

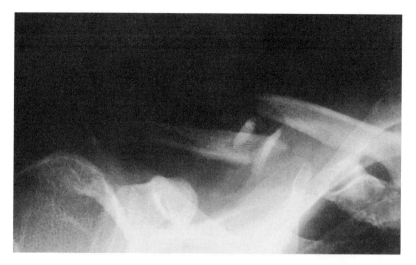

**Fig. 16-1.** A displaced clavicle fracture.

or shoulder. A clavicle fracture can also be secondary to a direct blow. The athlete will often come off the field supporting the arm by the forearm or elbow. The player is usually able to localize the pain precisely on the clavicle and often describes a "crack" or "snap" at the time of impact. Gentle palpation reveals crepitus and swelling directly over the clavicle. Active range of motion is significantly decreased. A careful distal neurovascular exam is done to rule out concomitant injury to the brachial plexus or adjacent blood vessels. The injured extremity should be placed in a sling and ice applied over the fracture.[2] The patient should be evaluated with radiographs, although these may be done at the completion of competition if no significant swelling or neurovascular symptoms or signs are present (Fig. 16-1). This may be a season-ending injury, and the patient should avoid athletic activity until clinical and radiographic union has occurred and until full strength and range of motion are restored. Often 12 to 16 weeks are required before an athlete can be returned to unlimited athletic participation.

## PROXIMAL HUMERUS FRACTURES

Fractures of the proximal humerus are uncommon in young athletes and are usually associated with significant trauma. The athlete complains of extreme pain in the shoulder (usually anterior). Physical examination reveals significant tenderness in the proximal humerus,

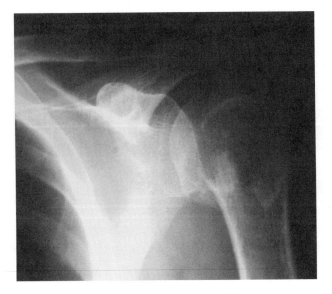

**Fig. 16-2.** A proximal humerus fracture.

and crepitation may be palpated. Active range of motion is extremely limited. With this clinical presentation, passive range-of-motion testing should be avoided. A careful neurovascular exam of the arm should be done. A sling and ice should be applied. The athlete should be evaluated with formal radiographs, but these may be done at the completion of the game if significant swelling or neurovascular compromise is absent (Fig. 16-2).

## SCAPULA FRACTURES

Scapula fractures are highly uncommon athletic injuries and are secondary to high-energy trauma applied to the posterior thorax. Scapula fractures are commonly associated with significant pulmonary or thoracic injuries.[6] Examination reveals severe pain over the scapula, with crepitation and swelling. Auscultation of the lungs and heart should be done to exclude concomitant injury. Careful palpation will often reveal fracture of multiple adjacent ribs. An athlete with a scapula fracture should be transferred immediately to the emergency room and evaluated for associated injuries to the thorax. If no other injuries are present, scapula injuries are treated symptomatically; the athlete is allowed to return to competition when pain-free, full range of motion and strength are obtained.

# INSTABILITY

Acute instability of the shoulder manifested by dislocations and subluxations is seen in both the acromioclavicular and glenohumeral joints. These injuries are more common in contact sports and are typically secondary to excessive force indirectly applied to the joint from the upper extremity.

## ACROMIOCLAVICULAR SEPARATIONS

Acromioclavicular separations represent a spectrum of injuries—from stretching of the ligaments without displacement, to displacement of the distal clavicle from the acromion. The integrity of the acromioclavicular joint is maintained by the acromioclavicular joint ligament and capsule and by the coracoclavicular ligaments—the conoid and trapezoid ligaments. The acromioclavicular joint capsule and ligaments primarily limit horizontal (anterior and posterior) translation, and the stronger coracoclavicular ligaments limit superior translation of the clavicle.[3] Disruption occurs sequentially, with stretching and tearing of the acromioclavicular joint ligaments followed by the stretching and tearing of the coracoclavicular ligament complex.

The mechanism of injury may be either a fall on the outstretched hand or, more commonly, a fall directly onto the shoulder—forcing the scapula and acromion away from the distal clavicle. The athlete will generally complain of pain on the top of the shoulder. Examination should be done after the jersey and shoulder pads are removed. The player can usually localize the tenderness to the acromioclavicular joint, although diffuse tenderness may be present in the trapezius and deltoid. Observation should allow one to distinguish between a nondisplaced distal clavicle (type I) and a displaced distal clavicle (type II or III)[1] (Fig. 16-3). Distinguishing between a type II injury with stretching of the coracoclavicular ligaments, and a type III injury with complete rupture of the ligaments, may be difficult on clinical examination. Comparison with the contralateral side and knowledge of the athlete's preparticipation exam are critical, as acromioclavicular separations are quite common among athletes who play contact sports and may represent an old injury. Palpation at the acromioclavicular joint should be done carefully and the joint assessed for anterior and posterior translation, as well as the more obvious superior translation. Active range of motion and strength should then be tested. Strength should be specifically tested with the arm in the cross-arm position (horizontally adducted across the body). With a subtle injury, the cross-arm position will also reproduce pain at the acromioclavicular joint itself. Displaced acromioclavicular separations (types II and III) generally present with significant weakness and decreased active

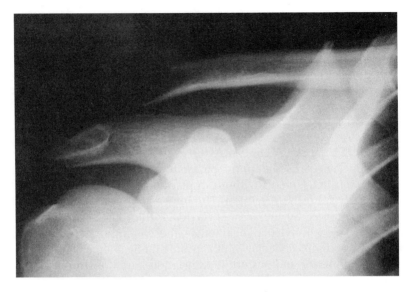

**Fig. 16-3.** A type III acromioclavicular separation.

range of motion. The injury should be treated with the application of ice and a supporting sling. Radiographic evaluation should be done at the completion of the competition. After a diagnosis is made, the athlete may be treated with functional rehabilitation. Return to play is allowed when full strength and active range of motion are present. Occasionally the athlete may be allowed to return to the game on the day of injury. Sport- and position-specific activities (e.g., throwing—for a quarterback or pitcher) must be assessed before the athlete is permitted to return.

An athlete participating in a contact sport may occasionally suffer a contusion of the acromioclavicular joint. This type of injury occurs secondary to a direct blow over the acromioclavicular joint itself and is seen most commonly in players with prominent acromioclavicular joints (check the contralateral side) and insufficient padding. The athlete notes pain and swelling directly over the acromioclavicular joint and often has less pain with movement and strength testing. This injury is treated like a type I injury, and the return-to-play criteria are the same. The athlete often benefits from a modification of protective padding before the next competition.

## GLENOHUMERAL INSTABILITY

Instability of the glenohumeral joint is a significant and potentially disabling injury. Most commonly, anterior instability—either subluxation or dislocation—is seen.[8] This injury occurs both in contact and noncontact sports. The mechanism of injury is generally excessive force placed on the

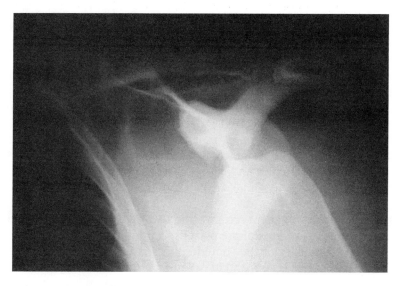

**Fig. 16-4.** An anterior shoulder dislocation.

abducted, externally rotated arm. The athlete with an anterior dislocation has severe pain in the shoulder and often states that the shoulder "popped out of joint." Observation of the shoulder with the jersey and pads removed reveals a squared-off shoulder with anterior fullness. Significant decrease in range of motion is noted both actively and with gentle, passive examination. A careful neurovascular examination must be done to rule out any associated injuries. If the neurovascular exam is normal and the shoulder is seen acutely, gentle internal and external rotation with distraction of the shoulder may reduce the dislocation. Excessive force should be avoided at all times. If the patient is not seen acutely (within 5 to 10 minutes) or if the shoulder dislocation is irreducible, the athlete should be transferred immediately to the hospital for radiographs and reduction. Reduction in this setting often requires intravenous analgesia and muscle relaxation. If reduction is accomplished on the field, the player should be placed in a sling or shoulder immobilizer, and ice should be applied to the shoulder. If the neurovascular exam remains intact, the athlete may be evaluated with radiographs at the end of competition. Radiographs should always include a good axillary or transthoracic view[7] (Fig. 16-4).

Anterior shoulder subluxation is a more subtle injury. The athlete complains of shoulder pain, but the range of motion is often near normal, although painful. Observation reveals no obvious asymmetry from the contralateral side. The mechanism of injury is again abduction and external rotation, and the athlete will often note that the shoulder "slipped out and back into place." Examination of the player will usually reveal significant apprehension when the injured arm is placed in the provocative externally rotated and abducted positions. The athlete should not be allowed to return to competition unless full, active range of motion and strength are present.

After radiographic evaluation and reduction (if necessary), anterior instability is usually addressed conservatively. After a short period of immobilization, a functional rehabilitation program (emphasizing dynamic stability of the shoulder) is initiated. When the athlete has full, pain-free range of motion and strength, a return to competition can be considered. The athlete should be carefully counseled about the risk of injury recurrence and possible need for surgery with the return to competition. Use of a shoulder brace or strap to limit abduction and external rotation can be considered if the player's sport and position allow.

Posterior instability of the shoulder is less common in athletes. True posterior dislocation is rare, and most athletes present with posterior subluxation. The position of risk with posterior subluxation is generally forward flexion and internal rotation with a posteriorly directed force applied to the arm and proximal humerus.[4] This is most commonly seen in football among offensive linemen. The athlete generally complains of the shoulder "slipping out the back." The player can often reproduce the position that causes the discomfort and will place the arm in the forward flexed and internally rotated position. Often the athlete admits to several previous episodes of this slipping. Physical examination often reveals posterior tenderness, apprehension when placed in the position of risk, and weakness of the external rotators of the shoulder. The athlete's shoulder should be iced and placed in a shoulder immobilizer, with the arm in neutral rotation (to avoid exacerbation of the internally rotated position). The athlete should be allowed to return to play only when full range of motion and strength are achieved. The athlete should be evaluated with radiographic studies, and a rehabilitation program emphasizing external rotation strength and dynamic stabilization should be initiated.

## ROTATOR CUFF INJURIES

The rotator cuff consists of four muscles: subscapularis, supraspinatus, infraspinatus, and teres minor. These muscles stabilize the humeral head in the glenoid and assist in the coordinated motion of the arm.

Rotator cuff injuries are common among athletes. An acute cuff injury is usually secondary to a forced stretch of the tendons and occurs most commonly in collision or contact sports. The mechanism is often forceful rotation or movement of the arm against resistance. This may occur as a single acute injury, or the athlete may complain of multiple small injuries to the shoulder.[5] The athlete complains of weakness of the shoulder with a variable amount of pain. The player is often unable to precisely localize the pain and notes its location as "deep" in the shoulder. Palpation usually reveals tenderness of the rotator cuff attachments to the humeral head. Strength testing will reveal variable deficits in cuff strength. Strength should be tested in external and internal rotation with the arm at the side (0 degrees of abduction) and with the empty can test. A careful neurovascular exam should be completed and the patient questioned regarding sensory changes or neck pain. This should be done to ensure the cuff dysfunction is secondary to direct injury to the cuff and not secondary to neurologic injury. Pain in the neck or trapezius, sensory deficits, or weakness in the deltoid suggests a neurologic lesion. The patient should be allowed to return to play only if full, active range of motion and normal strength are present. The presence of any neurologic abnormality (motor or sensory) is a contraindication to return to play until the abnormality has completely resolved. After the game has ended, the athlete should be evaluated with plain radiographs. Significant weakness at the rotator cuff should be evaluated with an MRI or arthrogram to delineate the integrity of the rotator cuff (Fig. 16-5). In a young athlete, a complete tear of the cuff that is accompanied by weakness should be considered for surgical repair. Rotator cuff strains should be treated with functional rehabilitation. Return to competition should be allowed when full, pain-free range of motion and strength are present.

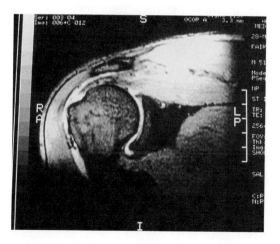

**Fig. 16-5.** Magnetic resonance imaging (MRI) of a full-thickness rotator cuff tear.

# CONTUSIONS

Contusions of the shoulder girdle are common and are seen most often in contact or collision sports. A contusion occurs secondary to a direct blow, and the player generally remembers being struck on the shoulder. Careful palpation will reveal the point of maximum tenderness, and the shoulder should be checked for evidence of a neurologic lesion or crepitation. The athlete should be allowed to return to play only if full, active range of motion and strength are demonstrated. If allowed by the sport and position, local padding can be applied to protect the injured part.

# MUSCULOTENDINOUS INJURIES

Musculotendinous injuries—other than to the rotator cuff, and most commonly to the pectoralis or deltoid—are occasionally seen in athletes. The athlete with such an injury has localized pain and generally describes a mechanism of injury with forced movement against resistance. A "tear" or "snap" is occasionally described by the player. An effort should be made to delineate the precise mechanism of injury sustained, as this often gives clues to the injured musculotendinous unit. Examination necessitates careful palpation to localize the point of maximum tenderness and the presence of swelling or ecchymosis. After the injured muscular tendon is identified, specific strength testing is done. An athlete with any significant weakness should be treated with ice and a sling. Full, active range of motion and strength should be present before return to play is allowed. Significant weakness is indicative of a complete tear, and further radiographic study (magnetic resonance imaging [MRI]) should be considered. Fortunately, complete ruptures are quite rare, and a functional rehabilitation program should be initiated as soon as possible.

### References

1. Allman FL Jr: Fractures and ligamentous injuries of the clavicle and its articulation, *J Bone Joint Surg* 19A:774-784, 1967.
2. Anderson K, Jensen P, Lauritcen J: Treatment of clavicular fractures: figure of eight bandage vs. a simple sling, *Acta Orthop Scand* 57:71-74, 1989.
3. Fukuda K, Craig EV, An KN et al: Biomechanical study of the ligamentous system of the acromioclavicular joint, *J Bone Joint Surg* 68A:434-439, 1986.
4. Hawkins RJ, Koppert G, Johnston G: Recurrent posterior instability (subluxation) of the shoulder, *J Bone Joint Surg* 66A:169-174, 1984.
5. Hill JA: Epidemiologic perspective on shoulder injuries, *Clin Sports Med* 2:241-245, 1983.
6. McGahan JP, Rab GT, Dublin A: Fractures of the scapula, *J Trauma* 20:880-883, 1980.
7. O'Brien SJ, Warren RF, Schwartz E: Anterior shoulder instability, *Orthop Clin North Am* 18:395-408, 1987.
8. Rowe CR: Prognosis in dislocations of the shoulder, *J Bone Joint Surg* 38A:957-977, 1956.

# Chapter 17

# Injuries to the elbow

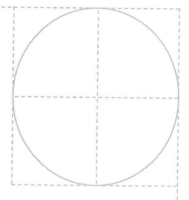

Laura A. Timmerman

## MECHANISM OF INJURY

Acute elbow injuries are usually the result of direct trauma. The most common injury mechanism is a fall on the outstretched arm. Other mechanisms include direct-contact injuries and noncontact throwing injuries. Chronic elbow problems are usually the result of overuse injuries from the repetitive microtrauma of throwing.

## CLINICAL DIAGNOSIS

### SUBJECTIVE

Initially, the mechanism of injury should be determined. The athlete should be asked whether he or she felt or heard a "pop" in the elbow. Activities that worsen or relieve the symptoms should be noted. For chronic injuries, any recent changes in training or throwing technique should be addressed. The location of the pain and the presence of neurologic symptoms, including sensory changes or motor weakness, are important in the history.

### OBJECTIVE
#### Skin

The skin should be inspected first for any evidence of lacerations or abrasions, which may indicate an open fracture. An open fracture is *a medical emergency* and necessitates operative treatment ideally within the first 6 hours of injury.

#### Neurovascular

The neurovascular structures are in close proximity to the elbow joint. Injuries to the nerves and vessels about the elbow can occur with trauma, especially elbow dislocations. It is crucial to document the on-field neurovascular exam at the time of injury. The distal radial pulse should be evaluated; to attempt to palpate the brachial pulse at the elbow may be too painful. If the radial artery is not palpable, the capillary refill of the fingertips can be compared with the other side. Any vascular deficit is a *medical emergency*, and the patient should be immediately transported to the nearest hospital.

The median, radial, and ulnar nerves all cross the elbow joint. The athlete with a median nerve deficit has weakness in the wrist flexors and finger flexors of the thumb, index, and long fingers and experiences sensory changes in the tips of these fingers. The athlete with an ulnar nerve deficit has weakness in the interossei muscles of the hand and with flexion of the distal interphalangeal joint of the little finger. The athlete with a radial nerve deficit has weakness in the wrist and finger extensor muscles and experiences sensory changes on the dorsum of the hand.

### Range of motion

The amount of active range of motion the patient can perform should be noted. Normal range of motion for the elbow is 0 to 150 degrees of flexion, with 70 to 80 degrees of pronation (turn palm down) and 80 to 90 degrees of supination (turn palm up).

### Palpation

Areas of crepitus and swelling should be noted, as well as the point of maximum tenderness. The location of tenderness is important in the dif-

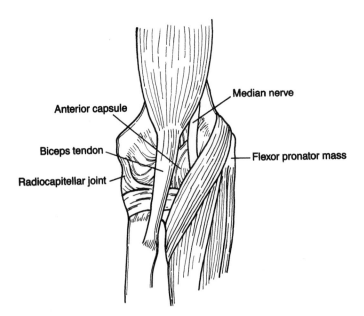

Median nerve

Anterior capsule

Biceps tendon

Flexor pronator mass

Radiocapitellar joint

**Fig. 17-1.** An anterior view of the elbow.

ferential diagnosis. The anterior, posterior, medial, and lateral aspects of the elbow should be examined (Figs. 17-1 to 17-4). Pain is present over the radiocapitellar joint with pronation and supination injury to this area. It is also very important to carefully examine the distal radioulnar joint for tenderness in order to rule out any injury that involves both the elbow and the wrist. In addition, the shoulder and cervical spine should be examined to rule out other injuries that could cause elbow pain.

**Strength**

The strength and integrity of the triceps, biceps, wrist flexors, and wrist extensors should be tested to rule out avulsion or tearing of these structures. Weakness may also indicate a nerve injury.

**Stability**

The stability of the elbow should be carefully assessed. Valgus stress, or placing a lateral stress on the forearm while the humerus is stabilized, is important in the evaluation of the medial ligaments. Varus stress (a medial stress applied to the forearm) should also be examined.

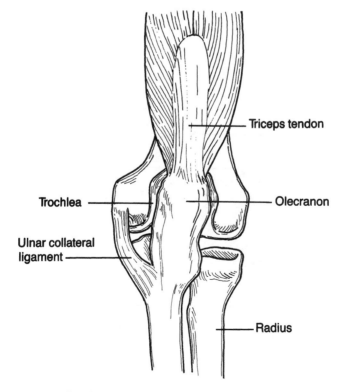

**Fig. 17-2.** A posterior view of the elbow.

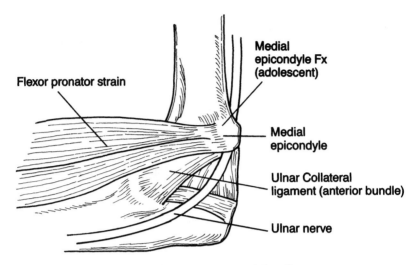

**Fig. 17-3.** A medial view of the elbow.

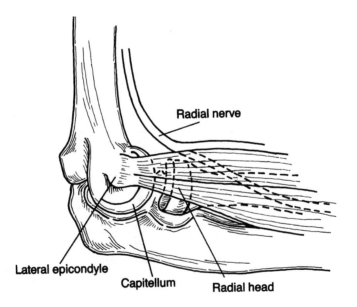

**Fig. 17-4.** A lateral view of the elbow.

# PERTINENT DIFFERENTIAL DIAGNOSIS

## FRACTURE-DISLOCATION

Fracture-dislocation is a relatively common athletic injury to the elbow. The athlete with this type of injury has a painful and swollen elbow and is resistant to any range of motion.

### Radial head fracture

A radial head fracture usually results from a fall on the arm. The athlete is tender laterally and has pain with pronation and supination.

### Olecranon fracture

An olecranon fracture results from direct trauma or a contraction of the triceps. The pain is located over the olecranon posteriorly.

### Dislocation

If the elbow is dislocated, the contour is abnormal, and the athlete is in a great deal of pain. A neurovascular exam is essential since this injury is associated with an increased incidence of neurovascular injury. A dislocation is also commonly associated with fractures of the radial head, the coronoid process of the ulna, or the humerus.

### Both-bone forearm fracture

A fall on the outstretched arm can result in fractures of both the radius and the ulna. The forearm appears deformed and is very painful to palpation. The neurovascular status should be carefully assessed.

### Medial epicondyle fracture

A medial epicondyle fracture is seen frequently among adolescent athletes, who can fracture across the open growth plate at the medial epicondyle. An athlete with this type of injury has tenderness and swelling over the medial epicondyle and has pain with motion of the elbow.

## ACUTE SOFT TISSUE INJURY

### Ulnar collateral ligament rupture

The ulnar collateral ligament is the main stabilizer to valgus stress at the elbow. The elbow is placed under tremendous valgus stress during throwing, and it can also suffer valgus stress if a force is applied across the forearm of an outstretched arm (e.g., when a baseman tags a runner or while a passing quarterback is tackled). This ligament usually tears as a result of repetitive microtrauma, but an acute rupture can occur. The player usually complains of pain in the medial side of the elbow; he or she may have heard a "pop" and may have ulnar nerve symptoms (pain and tingling down the forearm to the little finger). The elbow may be unstable to valgus stress testing. If the injury is severe, an acute medial rupture of the elbow—including the ulnar collateral ligament, the medial capsule, and the flexor-pronator mass—may have occurred.

**Biceps tendon rupture**

A biceps tendon rupture is usually a traumatic event and is more often seen in the older athlete (over 30 to 40 years old) who is involved in heavy lifting. It may be associated with steroid use. The athlete has pain in the antecubital fossa and weakness with supination and flexion. The biceps tendon may not be palpated, but this can be difficult to determine with swelling.

**Triceps tendon rupture**

A triceps tendon rupture results from a fall or direct blow to the elbow, or from contraction of the triceps. The athlete has posterior elbow pain and swelling, and there is weakness with active elbow extension. This injury can also be associated with an elbow dislocation.

**Anterior capsular strain**

The mechanism of injury for an anterior capsular strain is hyperextension of the elbow without dislocation. The player complains of anterior elbow pain, and there is pain with attempted extension of the elbow—which places a stretch on the anterior tissues. The biceps tendon should be carefully evaluated for injury.

**Compartment syndrome**

Compartment syndrome results after traumatic injury with swelling in a contained fascial compartment. The fascial compartments of the forearm may be affected, especially with fractures of the forearm bones, or after an elbow dislocation. The athlete complains of extreme pain and has pain with resisted passive extension or flexion of the fingers. The forearm may feel tight and be tender to palpation. Distal pulses may be affected, but they are usually normal. This is a *medical emergency*, and the athlete needs to be immediately transported to the hospital for evaluation and possible surgical release. Permanent neurologic injury can result with a prolonged increase in pressures.

**Loose body in the elbow joint**

The athlete may complain of locking and may describe a history of a "pop" or "catching" in the elbow joint. This is seen especially in the adolescent athlete. A loose osteochondral fragment can result—either from the breaking off of an osteophyte or from an osteochondritis dissecans lesion. The athlete exhibits swelling over the lateral "soft spot" of the elbow and may have a decrease in the range of motion of the joint.

## ON-FIELD TREATMENT

A careful physical examination should be performed on the athlete. If the athlete exhibits painful or restricted range of motion, a posterior splint should be applied. If there is an obvious deformity to the elbow or forearm, the splint can be applied and the athlete transferred to the local hospital. If the player is more than 45 to 60 minutes from a treatment facility, the arm should be anatomically approximated before transfer, especially if there is neurovascular compromise.

If the elbow is dislocated, radiographs before reduction are preferred. In certain situations, a reduction on the field may be necessary if the player is a prolonged (more than 60 minutes) distance from the hospital. The most common direction of elbow dislocation is posterior, with the forearm bones located posterior to the distal humerus. The simplest method of reduction is to have an assistant apply countertraction to the humerus while the trainer or physician applies distal traction by grasping the forearm and wrist. The medial or lateral displacement is corrected first, and then distal traction is applied as the elbow is flexed. Downward pressure on the forearm, or posterior pressure on the humerus, may be necessary to disengage the coronoid out of the olecranon fossa. Hyperextension should be avoided because of the danger of neurovascular injury. This reduction method should only be attempted in an urgent situation when a hospital is not in close proximity, and more than one attempt should be avoided. If the reduction is unsuccessful after one attempt, the athlete should be quickly transported to a center where intravenous sedation or a general anesthetic can be given.

**Posterior splint**

A posterior splint is a universal method of immobilization for the elbow joint. It is easily made from 5-inch plaster or fiberglass rolls, with padding applied to the inner layer. The material is placed behind the arm, extending from just below the axilla to the wrist. The arm is safely immobilized with the elbow flexed at 90 degrees, or in the position of comfort for the athlete. If casting material is unavailable, a pillow, cardboard box, or bulky towels can be placed around the arm for protection.

**Injections**

Injections about the elbow for acute injuries are not indicated in the on-field setting. In certain situations with chronic injuries, an injection—after conservative treatment has failed, and radiographs have been evaluated—may be indicated. Injections about the elbow can be associated with subsequent tendon and ligament injuries and should be approached with caution.

## GUIDELINES FOR NECESSARY FURTHER WORK-UP

Any injury that results in swelling, with pain and a restriction in range of motion, should be evaluated with initial radiographs of the elbow and a careful follow-up examination. Displaced fractures and soft tissue injuries may require surgical treatment. Once a diagnosis is confirmed, a treatment plan and rehabilitation program can be prescribed.

The evaluation of the injured elbow should be prompt because prolonged immobilization of the elbow can result in pain and stiffness that can be difficult to treat.

## RETURN-TO-PLAY CRITERIA

1. No joint effusion
2. No tenderness on examination
3. Normal strength and range of motion
4. No instability

Once the athlete has met the above criteria, then he or she should be started slowly back to activity before a return to full play. For example, the throwing athlete would require a progressive increase in the distance thrown with the use of an interval throwing program. Occasionally, after a contact injury to the elbow, an athlete returns to the sideline with a large hematoma over the elbow; he or she has full range of motion of the joint and normal strength without pain, and there is no evidence of intraarticular swelling. This athlete can be allowed to return to play and be reevaluated as necessary.

### Bibliography

American Academy of Orthopaedic Surgeons: Arm, elbow, and forearm. In *Athletic training and sports medicine*, ed 2, Rosemont, Ill, 1991, The Academy.

Andrews JR, Schemmel SP, Whiteside JA: Evaluation, treatment, and prevention of elbow injuries in throwing athletes. In Nicholas JA, Hershman EB, editors: *The upper extremity in sports medicine*, St Louis, 1990, Mosby–Year Book.

Hotchkiss RN, Green DP: Fracture dislocations of the elbow. In Rockwood CA Jr, Green DP, editors: *Fractures in adults*, ed 3, Philadelphia, 1991, JB Lippincott.

# Chapter 18

# Injuries to the hand and wrist

Keith Meister

The hand-wrist unit is one of the most commonly injured areas in athletics. Such is probably the case because the hand is characteristically held in front of the athlete in most sports and therefore frequently absorbs the initial contact. Fortunately, however, most of the injuries that do occur are not serious enough to necessitate restraint from athletic competition. A quick return to sport activity and avoidance of an adverse outcome are dependent on early accurate diagnosis, proper management of the problem, and often an innovative approach to splinting and protection of the injury. Ultimately the burden of clearing an athlete for return to play falls on the team or individual's treating physician.

## SPLINTING

In general, most athletes with injuries to the hand and wrist can at some point in the healing process be safely allowed back into competition with appropriate splinting and casting techniques. The types of materials allowed on the injured extremity, which provide for adequate protection and safe participation, vary from sport to sport and among various levels of athletic competition. On the college level, in football, the NCAA has very specific guidelines regarding illegal equipment, which includes the following materials:

> Art. 5b. Hard, abrasive or unyielding substances on the hand, wrist, forearm or elbow of any player, unless covered on all sides with closed-cell, slow-recovery foam padding no less than 1/2 inch thick or an alternate material of the same minimum thickness and similar physical properties. Hard or unyielding substances are permitted only to protect an injury, and hand and arm protectors (casts or splints) are permitted only to protect a fracture or dislocation.

However, in other collision and contact sports (i.e., basketball and volleyball) hard protection on the upper extremity (i.e., orthoplast and casting) is

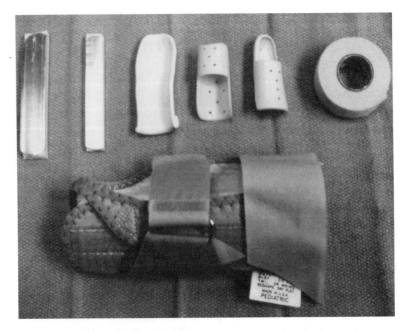

**Fig. 18-1.** Various splints used to protect the hand and wrist for early return of the athlete to competition.

generally not allowed by the referees. On a high school level allowable methods of splinting vary from state to state, and one should contact one's own high school athletic association to avoid any misinterpretation of the rules.

Mindful of such rules, a protective silicone rubber splint has been developed that works well at the wrist for protection of healing sprains or fractures. The splint is constructed with gauze impregnated with silicone rubber-RTV 11. Its use is exclusively for the purpose of protection during games and practice with the reapplication of a splint or cast at all other times. In the hand, varied taping techniques, buddy taping, and aluminum and stack splints can usually be used to safely protect and return most athletes to competition in the acute phases of healing (Fig. 18-1).

## THE WRIST

Most wrist injuries in athletics are caused by a fall onto an outstretched hand, with the wrist in a characteristically dorsiflexed position. Evaluation should begin with a recognition of the mechanism of injury,

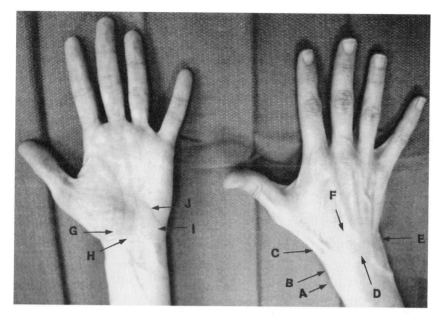

**Fig. 18-2.** The topographic anatomy of the wrist. Dorsal landmarks: *A,* distal radius; *B,* radial styloid; *C,* anatomic snuff-box; *D,* distal radioulnar joint; *E,* ulnar styloid; *F,* lunate. Volar landmarks: *G,* scaphoid tubercle; *H,* lunate; *I,* pisiform; *J,* hook of the hamate.

followed by the location, duration, intensity, and characteristics of the pain. Examination should begin with a quick evaluation of the entire upper extremity, specifically noting any obvious deformity.

A basic understanding of the topographic anatomy of the wrist is essential for arriving at an accurate initial diagnosis. Specifically, tenderness should be noted dorsally at the distal radius, radial styloid, anatomic snuff-box, distal radioulnar joint, ulnar styloid, triangular fibrocartilage complex (TFCC), and lunate (Fig. 18-2). Volarly, tenderness should be noted at the scaphoid tubercle, lunate, pisiform, and hook of the hamate (Fig. 18-2). Palpation with localization of all areas of tenderness; evaluation of range of motion; first active, followed by passive manipulation of the involved joints; and evaluation of grip and pinch strength should be performed. Athletes who have suspected fractures, dislocations, or severe intercarpal sprains (with some exceptions) should be removed from competition until adequate radiographic assessment has been performed. A standard radiographic profile of the wrist including a neutral posteroanterior view, anteroposterior or posteroanterior views in radial and ulnar deviation, and a true lateral view in neutral position should be obtained. Additional studies for further work-up may include magnetic resonance imaging (MRI), computed tomography (CT) scan, bone scan, tomograms, cineradiography, and arthrography.

## COMMON INJURIES TO THE WRIST
### Distal radioulnar joint dislocation
**Dorsal dislocation.** A dorsal dislocation of the distal radioulnar joint (DRUJ) occurs from a fall onto the outstretched wrist and forceful pronation of the forearm.

**Volar dislocation.** A volar dislocation of the DRUJ is less common; it occurs from a fall onto the outstretched wrist and forceful supination of the forearm.

**Diagnosis.** Swelling, dorsal or volar prominence of the ulnar head, and loss of forearm rotation with pain at the DRUJ are common. Radiographs and, if necessary, a CT scan can confirm the diagnosis.

**Treatment.** If an acute displacement is recognized at the time of injury, it may be treated with immediate manipulation. With dorsal dislocation, forceful supination of the wrist with pressure over the ulnar head will reduce the disruption. A long-arm cast with the forearm in full pronation should be applied.

With volar dislocation, forceful pronation of the wrist with pressure over the ulnar head will reduce the incongruity. A long-arm cast with the forearm in full pronation is then necessary. Radiographs or a CT scan is required to confirm concentric reduction. Occasionally surgery is needed to pin the joint in order to maintain a concentric reduction.

**Return-to-play criteria.** A period of 6 weeks of immobilization is necessary for complete healing. It is difficult for an athlete to return to competition before this point because of the necessity for long-arm cast immobilization.

### Distal radius fracture
A direct blow to the distal radius or a fall onto the outstretched hand with the wrist in dorsi- or volarflexion may cause a fracture.

**Diagnosis.** Swelling, possible deformity, tenderness about the distal radius, pain on range of motion of the forearm or wrist, and loss of grip strength are common. Radiographs can confirm the diagnosis.

**Treatment.** Ice and a volar wrist splint should be applied, and the athlete should be removed from competition. Nondisplaced, stable fractures necessitate 6 weeks of short-arm cast immobilization. Displaced and/or unstable fractures necessitate possible surgical intervention and long- and/or short-arm cast immobilization for 6 to 8 weeks.

**Return-to-play criteria.** Return to competition may be allowed following adequate treatment of the fracture and subsidence of the acute symptoms (with a stable fracture) after the first 1 to 2 weeks. Return to play is also dependent on whether adequate protection can be achieved through proper methods of splinting and casting. *Caution:* this determination is sports-specific and position-dependent!

**Ulnar styloid fracture**

A fall onto the outstretched hand with ulnar deviation of the wrist and direct trauma to the ulnar side of the wrist may cause an ulnar styloid fracture.

**Diagnosis.** Swelling, ulnar-side pain, tenderness over the ulnar styloid, and pain on ulnar deviation of the wrist are common. Radiographs can confirm the diagnosis.

**Differential diagnosis.** The differential diagnosis includes TFCC tears, lunatotriquetral sprains, and flexor carpi ulnaris (FCU) strains.

**Treatment.** A short-arm cast should be used, or a volar wrist splint should be applied for 4 to 6 weeks.

**Return-to-play criteria.** After confirmation of the diagnosis, the athlete may return—with proper splinting of the wrist—to contact sports. Heavy taping alone may not be sufficient to provide an adequate level of comfort or protection in the acute phases of healing.

**Triangular fibrocartilage complex injuries**

Tears of the TFCC usually occur from an ulnar blow to the hand, forcing the wrist into dorsiflexion and pronation. Tears may also occur while swinging a bat or racquet.

**Diagnosis.** Local tenderness at the DRUJ, a painful ulnar click or catch, and occasional distal radioulnar instability. Radiographs, arthrogram, and MRI (if necessary) can confirm the diagnosis.

**Differential diagnosis.** The differential diagnosis includes subluxation of the extensor carpi ulnaris, lunatotriquetral instability, pisotriquetral degeneration, and general ligamentous laxity.

**Treatment.** After a partial tear, an athlete can return to play with protective casting. A complete tear necessitates repair or excision, with appropriate casting and protection; return to competition is allowed upon the subsidence of acute symptoms. For sports that involve impact loading of the upper extremity, as well as racquet sports and baseball, the injury may have to heal completely (6 to 8 weeks) before the athlete can return to play.

**Ligamentous injuries and radiocarpal-lunate-perilunate dislocations**

A fall onto the outstretched hand, with the wrist usually dorsiflexed and a radial or ulnar load usually applied, can result in a ligamentous injury.

**Diagnosis.** Swelling, diffuse pain, and positive or negative deformity with dorsal or volar prominences may be noted. With volar dislocations, acute median and/or ulnar nerve compression symptoms are possible. Weakness of power grip is present. Wrist radiographs can confirm the diagnosis.

**Differential diagnosis.** The differential diagnosis includes minor radio- or ulnocarpal sprains to patterns of complete dislocation.

**Treatment.** Ice and a volar wrist splint should be applied to a suspected severe injury. Minor ligamentous injuries—characterized by minimal tenderness; full active and passive range of motion, with little pain elicited at the extremes of motion; and good power grip strength—may be taped, and the athlete may be immediately returned to competition. If symptoms persist, the athlete is removed from competition and radiographs should be obtained to rule out occult fractures and/or instability of the wrist.

Radiocarpal dislocations are often associated with fractures of the distal radius and necessitate surgical intervention. Isolated lunate or perilunate dislocations necessitate closed manipulation and oftentimes further surgical intervention. In the event that gross deformity of the wrist is encountered, it is usually best to obtain clear radiographs of the injury before attempting manipulation.

**Return-to-play criteria.** Immediate return to activity is allowed for an athlete who has a confirmed minor sprain of the wrist, provided that symptomatic splinting and heavy taping are used until full range of motion and strength are achieved. An athlete with a small avulsion fracture of the carpal bone, without major ligamentous injury, may return to competition if adequate protection can be provided in an appropriate volar splint or silicone cast. An athlete with a complex dislocation requires at least 4 weeks of cast immobilization following closed manipulation or surgery, with resumption of activity and wrist immobilization in a silicone cast for an additional 4 weeks.

### Scaphoid fracture (body or waist)

A fall onto the outstretched hand with the wrist dorsiflexed and slightly radially deviated can cause a scaphoid fracture.

**Diagnosis.** Dorsal swelling, tenderness in the anatomic snuff-box, pain on dorsiflexion or radial deviation, and radial wrist pain on power grip are common. Radiographic evaluation can confirm the diagnosis.

**Differential diagnosis.** The differential diagnosis includes a scaphoradial or intercarpal ligament sprain, a fracture of the distal radius or styloid, and a thumb carpometacarpal sprain.

**Treatment.** If a scaphoid fracture is highly suspected, the athlete should be removed from competition; ice and a radial gutter or volar wrist splint should be applied. If initial radiographs are negative and clinical suspicion is great, a short- or long-arm thumb spica cast should be applied; radiographs should be repeated at 10 to 14 days postinjury. Displaced fractures necessitate surgical management; nondisplaced fractures may be treated with a long- and/or short-arm thumb spica cast.

**Return-to-play criteria.** With negative radiographs an athlete may return to competition in an allowable, rigid, short-arm thumb spica orthosis or cast—until he or she is asymptomatic or until a negative bone scan is obtained. An athlete with a nondisplaced fracture may be allowed to return to contact sports in a rigid orthosis for games once the acuteness of the injury has subsided (usually 1 to 2 weeks). However, the risk for further injury and compromised healing should be carefully explained to the athlete, and clearance by the team physician is necessary before return to competition is allowed.

An athlete with a displaced fracture necessitating surgical management follows guidelines for return to play similar to those stated previously for an athlete with a suspected or nondisplaced fracture.

**Hook of hamate fracture**

A hook of hamate fracture results from a fall onto the outstretched hand with direct trauma to the hook; or (more commonly) this type of injury occurs during a tennis, baseball, or golf swing. The butt of the handle may strike the hook and fracture it, or a violent contraction of the FCU can pull through the pisohamate ligament and jerk the hook.

**Diagnosis.** Complaints of volar-ulnar–side pain, poor power grip, and tenderness over the hook are noted. Radiographic evaluation with a carpal tunnel view and supination obliques can confirm the diagnosis.

**Treatment.** Nondisplaced fractures and small fragments are treated with a short gauntlet cast for 3 to 6 weeks. Large displaced fragments are treated with excision.

**Return-to-play criteria.** Immediate return to play with a short gauntlet cast is possible in contact sports. It is usually 3 to 4 weeks at least, in both conservatively and operatively treated cases, before the athlete is able to swing a bat, club, or racquet.

# THE HAND

Injury to the hand, unlike injury to the wrist because of the tendency of the digits to protrude and get caught on equipment and clothing, is less likely to occur from a fall alone; rather, injury to the hand commonly occurs from a torsional load applied to a digit. The tendency for injuries of the hand to be viewed as even more trivial than those of the wrist is the primary factor resulting in an inexcusably less-than-optimal result.

Evaluation should note the mechanism of injury and the location, duration, intensity, and characteristics of the pain. Notation of any obvious deformity is a good clue as to the mechanism of injury and structures at risk for damage. As in the wrist, a basic understanding of topographic anatomy is essential for arriving at an accurate initial diagnosis. One should be familiar with the locations of the specific joints and their potential ligamentous and tendon attachments. Evaluation of digital range of motion—first active (isolating proximal interphalangeal [PIP] and distal interphalangeal [DIP] function), followed by passive motion (testing for joint stability and pinch and grip strength)—should be assessed. Evaluation of neurovascular status can be completed with a gross sensory examination and an assessment of capillary refill. Standard radiographs include anteroposterior and lateral views of the digit. The athlete with an injury to a digit can oftentimes continue to perform, with proper protection. Again, however, the ultimate burden of clearance for return to activity falls on the individual's private physician or team's medical coverage.

## THE THUMB

### CARPOMETACARPAL JOINT DISRUPTION (DISLOCATION OR FRACTURE-DISLOCATION): BENNETT'S FRACTURE

A hyperextension and/or hyperabduction injury across the volar aspect of the thumb metacarpal may result in isolated dislocation. Axial compression is usually necessary for the intraarticular fracture.

**Diagnosis.** Pain, swelling, crepitus, prominence at the base of the thumb metacarpal, and palpable instability are noted. Radiographs and stress radiographs can confirm the diagnosis.

**Treatment.** Isolated dislocation is a rare injury that necessitates concentric reduction for a successful outcome. Occasional pinning of the joint or even open ligamentous repair may be necessary. In either case, 6 weeks of immobilization is necessary for healing. Fracture-dislocations necessitate closed reduction and pinning in most cases, with 6 weeks of immobilization necessary for healing.

**Return-to-play criteria.** With either an isolated dislocation or a fracture-dislocation, return to contact sports may be allowed with proper application of a protective splint following treatment. This is not possible in the dominant extremity of a throwing or overhand athlete, or in activities involving weight bearing of the upper extremity.

### THUMB METACARPAL SHAFT FRACTURE

A somewhat uncommon injury, a thumb metacarpal shaft fracture usually occurs from an axially applied torsional force to the digit. Crepitus may be palpated with tenderness at the midshaft of the metacarpal. Closed reduction with possible pinning of the fracture is sometimes necessary; the player may return to contact athletics with a well-molded radial gutter splint.

## THUMB METACARPOPHALANGEAL JOINT DISLOCATION

A thumb metacarpophalangeal (MCP) joint dislocation results from forceful hyperextension of the MCP joint.

**Diagnosis.** Volar prominence of the metacarpal head, with dorsal orientation of the proximal phalanx, is noted. Dimpling of the palmar skin is usually an indication of a complex dislocation.

**Differential diagnosis.** The differential diagnosis includes a simple or complex dislocation with interposition of the volar plate between the metacarpal head and proximal phalanx.

**Treatment.** One should avoid longitudinal traction to the proximal phalanx, as this may convert a simple dislocation into an irreducible, complex dislocation. Force should be applied against the dorsal surface of the proximal phalanx, and a counter push should be applied against the metacarpal head. Immobilization is then maintained in a radial plaster splint for 2 weeks with continued protection until full, painless range of motion and strength are regained. Following an unsuccessful attempt at immediate closed reduction, radiographs should be obtained.

**Return-to-play criteria.** Competition may be resumed immediately—with the athlete using a silicone thumb spica splint; or (if properly applied) taping can be used to stabilize the thumb.

## ULNAR COLLATERAL LIGAMENT INJURY (SKIER'S THUMB)

Forced abduction of the thumb results in tearing of the ulnar collateral ligament (UCL).

**Diagnosis.** Swelling about the ulnar border of the thumb proximal phalanx, as well as tenderness over the UCL, is noted. An evaluation of stability, with a valgus stress applied to both the extended and the flexed joint, should be conducted. The opposite thumb may be used for comparison. Stress radiographs can confirm the diagnosis. Complete tears are characterized by a joint opening of greater than 30 degrees.

**Treatment.** Partial tears can be treated with thumb spica splint immobilization for 3 weeks. Most complete tears necessitate surgical repair of the ligament followed by 6 weeks of protection.

**Return-to-play criteria.** With either a partial or complete tear, an immediate return to competition can be possible with adequate taping of the thumb MCP joint and either application of a "clincher" strap (Fig. 18-3) or taping of the thumb into the palm of the hand.

Tears of the radial collateral ligament are far less common than tears of the UCL but are seen most often in volleyball players. An athlete with this injury may be allowed to return to competition immediately, with 3 to 6 weeks of protective splinting and/or taping.

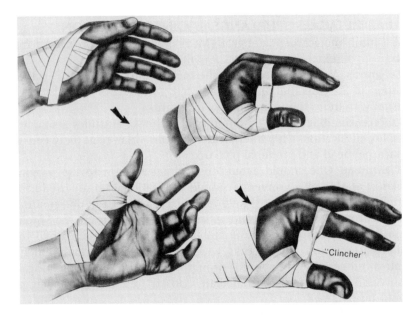

**Fig. 18-3.** The "clincher" strap taping technique for an ulnar collateral ligament (UCL) sprain of the thumb. (Illustrated by Ronald J. Ervin, B.F.A., AMI, Charllotesville, Va. With permission from Kulund DN: *The injured athlete,* Philadelphia, 1988, JB Lippincott.)

## THE FINGERS

Most injuries to the metacarpals, phalanges, and joints of the fingers of the hand are a result of torsional, abduction, and axial loads. Occasionally a crushing blow may be delivered that results in injury.

### METACARPAL FRACTURES
Metacarpal fractures occur most commonly in the fourth and fifth metacarpals.

**Diagnosis.** Dorsal swelling of the hand, loss of prominence of the metacarpal head, palpable crepitus or mobile fragments, and malrotation of the digits are common. Radiographs can confirm the diagnosis.

**Treatment.** Immediate care can be rendered with application of a volar splint and buddy taping of the involved digit to the adjacent digit. Multiple shaft fractures necessitate fixation, as do displaced intraarticular fractures at either end of the bone. Isolated fractures necessitate immobilization following reduction for at least 4 weeks. In contact sports, protection is best afforded for an additional 2 weeks with foam padding and buddy taping of the affected digit.

**Return-to-play criteria.** An individual may return to contact sports if an adequate, allowable splint can be fashioned for protection of the injury. This is not usually possible at the high school level. Therefore it is generally 4 weeks before return to play can occur, with protective buddy taping and padding necessary for an additional 2 weeks.

## METACARPOPHALANGEAL JOINT DISLOCATIONS

An MCP joint dislocation is usually a hyperextension injury. It most commonly occurs in the index finger.

**Diagnosis.** Swelling and deformity of the joint, with prominence of the metacarpal head in the palm, are noted. Dimpling of the skin at the midpalmar crease is usually indicative of entrapment of the volar plate.

**Treatment.** Immediate reduction should be done, with extension of the digit and pushing of the proximal phalanx volarward with a counterforce applied to the metacarpal head. *Do not apply longitudinal traction.* After an initial unsuccessful attempt at reduction, further attempts should be avoided. Oftentimes open reduction is necessary.

**Return-to-play criteria.** If a stable reduction is obtained, an individual can safely return to the game with buddy taping to the adjacent digit (if comfort and joint stability allow). A splinting program should be maintained for the first 3 weeks postinjury when the athlete is not in competition.

## PHALANGEAL FRACTURES (PROXIMAL-MIDDLE)

**Diagnosis.** Swelling and deformity of the digit, as well as tenderness at the shaft and palpable crepitus over the fracture site, are noted.

**Treatment.** Closed reduction or improved alignment of the fracture can usually be obtained with longitudinal traction and some degree of flexion or extension of the fragments. An appropriately fashioned dorsal aluminum splint with buddy taping to the adjacent digit is adequate protection until appropriate radiographs can be obtained. Many nondisplaced fractures can be treated with splinting alone. However, displaced, intraarticular, and unstable fractures will often necessitate reduction (either open or closed) and some form of internal fixation.

**Return-to-play criteria.** Adequate splinting and protection of the fracture can usually be obtained with a dorsal aluminum splint and buddy taping to the adjacent digit, with return to competition possible in the first 1 to 2 weeks postinjury. Fractures of the proximal phalanx may necessitate extension of the splint or taping below the MCP joint.

## PROXIMAL INTERPHALANGEAL JOINT INJURIES

Injuries to the PIP joint include articular fractures, fracture-dislocations, dislocations, collateral ligament injuries, and volar plate injuries.

### Dorsal dislocations

**Diagnosis.** Dorsal prominence of the proximal portion of the middle phalanx, with possible radial or ulnar deviation to the distal portion of the digit, is noted. Radiographs should be obtained to rule out concomitant fracture.

**Treatment.** Reduction with slight extension of the distal fragment should be done, followed by longitudinal traction and flexion to reduce the digit. The joint should then be reassessed for active motion and stability. The joint should be immobilized in about 30 degrees of flexion with a dorsal aluminum splint for 7 to 10 days. Buddy taping with active motion should then proceed for an additional 4 to 5 weeks. Return to competition may be allowed immediately, with splinting and buddy taping, if a congruent reduction of the joint is obtained.

**Lateral dislocation**

**Diagnosis.** Radial or ulnar deviation of the digit at the PIP joint is noted.

**Treatment.** Reduction with longitudinal traction should be done, followed by a reassessment of joint stability and active range of motion. A concentric reduction may be treated with splinting in 30 degrees of flexion for 3 weeks, followed by buddy taping and active range of motion for an additional 3 weeks. Follow-up radiographs should be obtained. Note that chronic instability as a late sequela is not an uncommon problem.

**Return-to-play criteria.** The athlete may return to competition immediately after reduction, with splinting and taping.

**Volar dislocation**

**Diagnosis.** Dorsal prominence of the head of the proximal phalanx is noted.

**Treatment.** Reduction—with slight flexion of the joint, longitudinal traction, and extension—should be done. Immobilization in full extension is necessary for 6 to 8 weeks. During competition protection is necessary for an additional 6 to 8 weeks. The MCP and DIP joints, however, may be left free to move.

**Return-to-play criteria.** The athlete may return to competition immediately, with concentric reduction and adequate splinting and buddy taping of the digit. Follow-up radiographs should be obtained to rule out intraarticular fracture.

*Note:* The inability to maintain a reduction may indicate a significant intraarticular fracture. However, if alignment can be maintained in a splint, competition may be resumed if the individual is both willing and comfortably able to play. Radiographs should be obtained following the event.

## PROXIMAL INTERPHALANGEAL SPRAINS

Injuries to the PIP joint may occur without fracture or actual dislocation. Isolated collateral ligament injuries should be diagnosed on routine stress evaluation of the injured joint. Treatment necessitates protective splinting of the joint in a position of slight flexion (30 degrees) for 7 to 10 days. Buddy taping should be used for protection during competition until full, active, painless motion is achieved.

Significant hyperextension to the joint without dislocation can cause injury to the volar plate. A painful PIP joint with tenderness at the volar plate should be treated with extension splinting until full, active, painless extension is achieved. Loss of extension following injury to the volar plate can lead to a late "pseudoboutoniere" deformity. Return to competition may be immediate.

## INJURIES TO THE DISTAL PHALANX AND DISTAL INTERPHALANGEAL JOINT

Most injuries to the distal tip of the finger occur as a result of a direct blow.

### Dislocations

Although they can occur volarly, most dislocations occur dorsally. Reduction can be achieved by first increasing the deformity, applying traction, and then performing reduction. Full, active range of the joint should be noted and dorsal aluminum or stack splinting used for at least 3 weeks or until full, painless range of motion is regained.

### Fractures

Pain, swelling, and ecchymosis of the distal phalanx after a blow to the tip of the finger may indicate a fracture. Full, active range of motion should be confirmed with protection of the digit in either a stack splint or aluminum splint curled over the tip of the digit before return to competition. Proper radiographs should be obtained following the event.

### Mallet finger

Injury to the tip of a digit may result in damage to the extensor mechanism. This is particularly common among baseball catchers and fielders, football receivers, and basketball players. Examination reveals loss of active extension-hyperextension of the joint. Treatment necessitates fulltime dorsal aluminum or stack splinting for 8 weeks in pure tendon injuries. On occasion, fixation of the DIP joint in extension with a buried wire across the joint is used for the period of healing, rather than a splinting program. Return to competition may be immediate with proper splinting, but radiographs should be obtained immediately following competition. Displaced fractures necessitate operative management, with return to competition allowed following appropriate treatment.

### Avulsion of the flexor digitorum profundus ("jersey finger")

Avulsion of the flexor digitorum profundus most commonly occurs to the ring finger of a football player while the athlete is grabbing an opponent's jersey. The ring finger gets caught up in the jersey and is forcibly extended against active flexion of the finger. Examination reveals an inability to actively flex the DIP joint of the affected digit. Tenderness is present on the volar aspect of the digit or even into the palm, depending on the level of retraction of the tendon. Treatment necessitates repair of the avulsed tendon, with protection of the digit for at least 6 weeks and a delay in return to competition for a similar period of time.

## NAIL BED INJURIES

Crush injuries or fractures to the distal portion of the digit can result in significant injury to the nail bed. These injuries are often marked by a significant subungual hematoma. A large collection of blood under the nail plate may be a sign of damage to the nail bed. The immediate treatment for a painful hematoma is evacuation. This can be effectively carried out with the "time honored" red-hot paper clip or the battery-operated cautery. An appropriate splint can then be applied for protection of the distal tip, and play can be resumed. If the individual is able to safely return to play following the injury, appropriate radiographs should be obtained after competition.

If the nail is lost or crushed, it is highly likely that the bed is significantly damaged and necessitates repair to avoid permanent deformity to the nail. A sterile dressing should be applied and the individual appropriately referred for further evaluation.

## CONCLUSION

Injuries to the hand and wrist are among the most common in sports. However, and fortunately, a correct initial evaluation can lead to a speedy return to athletics if appropriate diagnosis and management are rendered on the sideline. An aggressive (but not cavalier) approach to most problems may be used, keeping in mind the caveat to *always*—if in doubt over the safety of an individual's return—hold the athlete out!

### Bibliography

Adams JR: *NCAA football: rules and interpretation*, 1993.

Bassett FH: A protective splint of silicone rubber, *Amer J Sports Med* 7:358-360, 1979.

Culver JE: Sports-related fractures of the hand and wrist, *Clin Sports Med* 9:85-109, 1990.

Green DP: *Operative hand surgery*, ed 2, New York, 1988, Churchill Livingstone.

McCue FC: The elbow, wrist and hand. In Kulund DN, editor: *The injured athlete*, Philadelphia, 1988, JB Lippincott.

McCue FC, Mayer V: Rehabilitation of common athletic injuries of the hand and wrist, *Clin Sports Med* 8:731-776, 1989.

O'Brien ET: Acute fractures and dislocations of the carpus, *Orthop Clin North Am* 15:237-258, 1984.

Ruby LK: Common hand injuries in the athlete, *Orthop Clin North Am* 11:819-839, 1980.

# Chapter 19

# Contusions, abrasions, and lacerations

Kimberly Morris Fagan

Soft tissue injuries are frequent occurrences in sports. The majority are minor and necessitate little, if any, intervention. More significant soft tissue injuries occur and, if not recognized and treated appropriately, can result in long-term sequelae.

## CONTUSIONS

Contusions result from blunt trauma to soft tissue or bone. This leads to hematoma formation. The hematoma can be interstitial, intermuscular, or subperiosteal. Injuries are typically graded based on the degree of pain, swelling, and limitation of range of motion of the affected muscle group. Treatment principles are initially the same regardless of degree or location. These include rest, ice, compression, and elevation (RICE). Specific injuries are seen frequently in contact sports and are worth addressing on an individual basis.

### QUADRICEPS FEMORIS CONTUSIONS

A quadriceps femoris contusion results from a direct blow to the thigh. The resultant hemorrhage is near the intermuscular septum or fascial sheath (intermuscular) or within the muscle itself (intramuscular). The intermuscular hematoma initially may appear severe because of bruising associated with rapid tracking of the extravasated blood. It typically resolves rapidly. An intramuscular hematoma does not disperse as readily since the hemorrhage is confined within the muscle mass. Recovery, especially of range of motion, is slower.

The severity of a contusion is often unappreciated. After sustaining the injury and recovering from the initial pain of the blow, the athlete may continue to play. Only after significant bleeding and associated muscle spasms does the athlete note debilitating symptoms. These primarily include pain, swelling, and decreased range of motion.

Sideline evaluation reveals localized tenderness to palpation. In severe cases, especially if intramuscular in nature, a mass may be palpable. The quadriceps girth is documented to monitor the extent of swelling. Decreased knee flexion, secondary to pain and swelling, is noted. A sympathetic knee effusion may develop within the first 24 hours. Grading of a quadriceps contusion is based on limitation of range of motion as documented the day following the injury (Table 10).

Once a quadriceps contusion is recognized, treatment should begin immediately. Stage I of treatment focuses on controlling the hemorrhage. The player is removed from the game and the RICE protocol is implemented. Compression is achieved by flexing the hip to 90 degrees and flexing the knee as far as possible. This position is secured by wrapping an Ace bandage snugly around the thigh and lower leg. Ice is applied for 20 minutes at 20-minute intervals for the first several hours. Once the quadriceps girth has stabilized and the athlete is pain-free at rest, stage II of the treatment protocol is initiated.

Stage II focuses on recovery of pain-free range of motion. Ice is continued and nonsteroidal antiinflammatories are given to help control inflammation. Therapy focuses on gravity-assisted flexion with progression to active flexion and extension as tolerated. Once the athlete is pain-free at greater than 120 degrees of active flexion, with good quadriceps control noted, advancement to stage III is undertaken.

Stage III focuses on strength and functional capacity. Walking, light jogging, and swimming are acceptable in this stage. Once full, active, pain-free range of motion is obtained and functional drills are performed without pain, the athlete is returned to full activity. A recommendation should be made to the athlete to wear a thigh girdle with thick padding for the next 3 to 6 months for all contact sports.

Although rare, complications from quadriceps contusions do occur. Bleeding and edema in the anterior compartment of the thigh can be sig-

**Table 10**
**QUADRICEPS CONTUSION GRADING**

| Grade | Knee flexion |
| --- | --- |
| Mild | > 90° |
| Moderate | 45°-90° |
| Severe | < 45° |

nificant enough to lead to an acute compartment syndrome. Pain that seems out of proportion with clinical findings is the first clue. Sensory deficits may also occur. Once loss of pulses or motor deficits occur, the potential for irreversible damage is imminent or has already occurred. Diagnosis is made by documenting elevated compartment pressures. Once the diagnosis is established, a fasciotomy of the anterior compartment is performed. A high index of suspicion is necessary to prevent permanent disability.

Myositis ossificans refers to the development of ossification within the muscle. It occurs as a delayed complication of a quadriceps contusion. The more severe the initial injury, the higher the potential for complications. This diagnosis should be considered if a decrease in range of motion or an increase in pain is noted during therapy. Also, the development of a firm, palpable mass at the site of injury should prompt further investigation. The first radiographic signs may occur at 3 to 6 weeks postinjury. Complete maturation of the heterotrophic mass takes months. Treatment is usually conservative and successful. A rare individual with persistent pain and loss of function may require surgical excision. If surgery is attempted too early (i.e., before heterotrophic bone maturation), recurrence is common.

## HIP POINTERS

Hip pointer is a nonspecific term used to describe an injury resulting from a direct blow to the iliac crest. A contusion with soft tissue bleeding and swelling is the common pathologic condition. Iliac apophysitis or avulsion may less accurately be described as a hip pointer.

The athlete has localized pain, swelling, and decreased range of motion in the hip following a blow. The athlete typically has difficulty walking secondary to pain. Numerous muscles attach to the iliac crest. (See the box on p. 250.) The use of these muscles in rotation of the trunk and flexion of the hip causes pain.

Treatment is initiated with compression and relative rest. Crutches may initially be necessary. Ice and nonsteroidal antiinflammatories are useful in controlling inflammation. After the acute swelling and pain have abated, general stretching exercises are initiated. As these become pain-free, strengthening exercises follow. Return to activity is gradual, with pain serving as the primary guide. When the individual is ready to return to play, padding can provide some protection from direct contact.

## TACKLER'S ARM

"Tackler's" arm, or blocker's exostosis, is a bony prominence off the lateral aspect of the humerus. This results from a significant blow to the

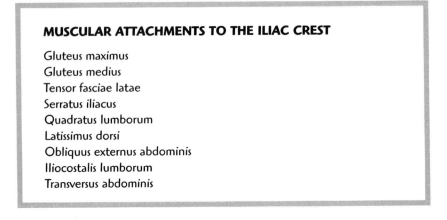

**MUSCULAR ATTACHMENTS TO THE ILIAC CREST**

Gluteus maximus
Gluteus medius
Tensor fasciae latae
Serratus iliacus
Quadratus lumborum
Latissimus dorsi
Obliquus externus abdominis
Iliocostalis lumborum
Transversus abdominis

unprotected arm or from multiple lesser hits to the same area. Pain and tenderness over the bony prominence are typical. Protective padding is usually sufficient. Rarely is surgical excision necessary.

## ABRASIONS

An abrasion is an area of body surface denuded of skin or mucous membrane by some unusual or abnormal mechanical process. In sports this typically occurs as a result of friction between a rough surface and the skin. Sliding into base, as in softball or baseball, with a resultant "strawberry" is a classic example. Diagnosis is straightforward. The affected area is denuded of skin with serous oozing noted.

Initial treatment includes adequate cleansing with hydrogen peroxide, soap and water, or an antibiotic scrub. A soft brush may be necessary to adequately remove any debris. Application of an antibiotic ointment to the affected area is advised. This should be covered by a nonadhesive type of dressing. The dressing should be changed daily, with the wound cleansed and antibiotic ointment reapplied until healing has occurred. Better results and pain relief may be achieved with the use of an occlusive, hydrocolloid dressing (i.e., Duoderm). This prevents scab formation and allows for reepithelialization at a faster rate. The dressing is replaced as needed.

Complications can occur with abrasions. If the wound is not adequately cleansed or appropriately cared for, a secondary bacterial infection may occur. This is denoted by inflammation of the surrounding tissue or by pustulant drainage from the affected area. Inadequate cleansing can also lead to "tattooing." This is a result of foreign material or dirt incorporating itself into the healing tissue.

# LACERATIONS

A torn, ragged, mangled wound is referred to as a laceration. This results from a direct blow over a bony prominence or from direct contact with a sharp or pointed object. The severity of bleeding and surrounding tissue trauma varies widely.

Control of bleeding is the first goal in laceration management. Application of gentle pressure to the blood source generally suffices. Wound exploration, cleansing, and debridement follow. Local anesthesia is often necessary before this can be accomplished.

Lidocaine (1%) is typically the agent of choice. Lidocaine with epinephrine (1:100,000 mg/ml or 1:200,000 mg/ml) is used for local anesthesia of facial lacerations. The epinephrine serves to control bleeding by vasoconstriction of the subdermal plexus. To avoid vascular compromise, lidocaine (1%) without epinephrine is used for lacerations involving the digits, nose, ears, or penis. The maximum dose of lidocaine with epinephrine is 3.5 mg/lb. The maximum dose of lidocaine without epinephrine is 2 mg/lb. Adverse reactions are rare if the recommended dose is not exceeded. If toxicity occurs it is initially manifested as nervousness, dizziness, or perioral tingling. In more severe cases convulsions, coma, or respiratory or cardiac arrest may occur.

Once adequate anesthesia is obtained, a thorough cleansing using normal saline irrigation is initiated. Removal of all dirt and debris is essential to prevent infection and delayed wound healing. Exploration of the wound is a standard part of cleansing. The identification of underlying vascular, tendon, or nerve injuries is necessary to appropriately manage the wound. Debridement of devitalized tissue may be necessary. Any jagged or beveled edges necessitate sharp, smooth debridement to allow for close approximation of wound edges—with resultant improved healing and decreased scar formation.

Simple lacerations not extending through the epidermis are adequately managed by reapproximation of skin edges using steristrips or butterflies. Lacerations extending through the epidermis generally necessitate suturing for adequate healing. A simple interrupted suture technique is used. Care should be taken to provide close skin-edge approximation without undue tension. Typically, nonabsorbable suture material is used. In cases involving the face, where cosmetic concerns are of importance, 5-0 to 7-0 nylon is used. For lacerations to the scalp and trunk the larger 3-0 to 4-0 nylon may be preferred. If the wound extends into or through the dermis, layered closure is necessary to obliterate dead space and allow for adequate reapproximation (while avoiding excess tension). Generally a 3-0 to 4-0 absorbable suture is recommended for deep closure. Cuticular sutures are then used to reapproximate the skin edges. Fortification of all laceration repairs is accomplished with adhesive strips. An antibiotic ointment is applied and is covered with an appropriate dressing. The wound should be kept dry for at least 24 hours.

Certain lacerations should not be closed. Because of the potential for infection it is generally recommended that a laceration should not be reapproximated more than 8 hours from the time of injury. An exception is sometimes made for facial lacerations up to 24 hours from time of injury. Human and animal bite wounds should not be sutured because of the high rate of contamination. Likewise, puncture wounds are left unsutured.

Suture removal varies depending on the location of the wound (Table 11). The longer they are left in place, the more scarring sutures produce.

**Table 11**
**TIMING OF SUTURE REMOVAL**

| Location of wound | Period of time |
|---|---|
| Face or neck | 3-4 days |
| Extremities | 5-8 days |
| Scalp or trunk | 7-10 days |

**Table 12**
**LACERATIONS THAT WARRANT SPECIAL CONSIDERATIONS**

| Affected area | Consideration |
|---|---|
| Eyebrow | Do not shave the eyebrow because it may grow back irregularly or not at all. |
| Eyelid | Consider an ocular injury, especially if full thickness is present. |
| Ear | Do not suture cartilage because of the risk of chondritis. |
| Lip | Meticulous reapproximation is necessary, particularly if the laceration crosses the vermilion border. |
| Cheek | Beware of a possible facial nerve or parotid duct injury. |

Certain lacerations necessitate referral to a specialist. Any athlete with a wound that has associated vascular, tendon, or nerve injury—or one that might necessitate future surgical revision—should be referred. Also, any request by a patient for a plastic surgeon should be honored. Special consideration must be given to particular lacerations (Table 12). If the primary caregiver feels uncomfortable with any laceration, the athlete should be referred to a physician more experienced in suturing techniques. Infection complicates the healing of a wound. It can result from inadequate cleansing, failure to remove a foreign body, or poor wound care following suturing. Any swelling, warmth, erythema, or persistent drainage should alert one to the possibility of infection. Antibiotic coverage should be initiated immediately. Suture removal with adequate debridement—followed by packing, where appropriate—is necessary. The wound will heal secondarily. Note that if a wound has a high potential for contamination, use of prophylactic antibiotics for 7 to 10 days is recommended. Polymicrobial coverage is necessary—with a first-generation cephalosporin, macrolide (e.g., erythromycin), or amoxicillin-clavulanate typically recommended.

Tetanus or lockjaw is a concern with contaminated wounds. Primary immunization is covered during the typical childhood vaccination series. Unfortunately, immunization records are often not available or childhood vaccinations were not initiated or completed. A primary vaccination series consists of two doses of 0.5 ml of absorbed tetanus-diphtheria toxoid (Td) given intramuscularly at least 4 weeks apart. The third dose is given 6 to 12 months following the second to complete the series. Once all three doses have been received a booster of Td is required at 10-year intervals to maintain adequate immunization status. Guidelines for tetanus prophylaxis in

**Table 13**
**GUIDELINES FOR TETANUS PROPHYLAXIS IN WOUND MANAGEMENT**

|  | Clean | Dirty |
|---|---|---|
| **Previously immunized** | | |
| Booster < 5 yrs | — | — |
| Booster 5-10 yrs | — | Td |
| Booster > 10 yrs | Td | Td |
| **Uncertain or unknown immunization status** | Td | Td and TIg |

*Td*, Tetanus-diphtheria toxoid; *TIg*, tetanus immunoglobulin.

wound management are based on immunization status and the potential of the wound for contamination (Table 13). A dirty wound is one that is obviously contaminated, greater than 24 hours old, frost bitten, or punctured. In cases in which tetanus immunoglobulin (TIg) is given, the dose is 250 U intramuscularly. If both Td and TIg are indicated, separate syringes and injection sites are advised. This prevents deactivation of Td by TIg.

## CONCLUSION

Contusions, abrasions, and lacerations are common occurrences in sports. Fortunately, if treated in an appropriate and timely manner, long-term sequelae are unlikely.

### Bibliography

American College of Physicians Task Force on Adult Immunization and Infectious Diseases Society of America: *Guide for adult immunization,* ed 3, Philadelphia, 1994, The College.

Amundson LH: Managing skin problems in athletes. In Melton MB, Walsh WM, Shelton GL, editors: *The team physician's handbook,* St Louis, Mosby–Year Book.

Arnheim DD, Prentice WE: *Principles of athletic training,* ed 8, St Louis, 1993, Mosby–Year Book.

Booher JM, Thibodeau GA: *Athletic injury assessment,* ed 3, St Louis, 1994, Mosby–Year Book.

Brunet ME, Hontas RB: The thigh, *Orthop Sports Med Princip Pract* 21:1086-1112, 1994.

Codner MA, Jones G: Repair techniques for facial wounds, *Emerg Med* 26:27-32, 1994.

Gomella LG et al: Suturing techniques. In Gomella LG, Braen GR, Olding MJ, editors: *Clinician's pocket reference,* ed 4, Garden Grove, Calif, 1983, Capistrano Press.

Harward MP: Adult immunizations: are you and your patients up-to-date? *Office-based Patient Encounters* 14:1016, 1993.

Reid DC: Injuries to the head and face. In Reid DC, editor: *Sports injury assessment and rehabilitation,* New York, 1992, Churchill Livingstone.

Reid DC: Soft tissue injuries of the thigh. In Reid DC, editor: *Sports injury assessment and rehabilitation,* New York, 1992, Churchill Livingstone.

Ryan JB et al: Quadriceps contusions: West Point update, *Am J Sports Med* 19:299-303, 1991.

Sanford JP: *Guide to antimicrobial therapy 1996,* Dallas, 1996, Antimicrobial Therapy.

# Appendix

# Running program

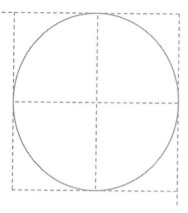

The following running program should be used as a measure of an athlete's progress as he or she returns from an injury to a lower extremity. When the athlete has completed the *entire* program, he or she is ready to return to competition.

The athlete may begin the running program when he or she can hop up and down on the toes of the injured extremity, without bearing weight on the other leg, 5 times.

## OUTDOORS

1. Jog 1 mile; stop immediately if you begin limping or if you have mild pain. When you can jog 1 mile pain free,*
   a. Do six 80-yard sprints at half speed. If you experience no pain or limping,
   b. Do six 80-yard sprints at three-quarter speed. If you experience no pain or limping,
   c. Do six 80-yard sprints at full speed. If you have no pain,
   d. Do six 80-yard cuts at three-quarter speed. If you have no pain,
   e. Do six 80-yard cuts at full speed. Always plant on the outside foot to cut. If you have no pain,

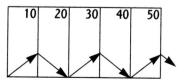

---

*If you do not complete the entire program on a particular day, start at the beginning the following day.

2. Do 10 minutes of running and/or jumping drills related to your sport. When you have completed the entire running program, you are ready to return to competition.*

## INDOORS

1. Jog 18 laps around the basketball court. Stop immediately if you begin limping or if you have mild pain. If you are pain free,†
   a. Do 15 lengths of the gym at half speed. If you have no pain,
   b. Do 15 lengths of the gym at three-quarter speed. If you have no pain,
   c. Do 15 lengths of the gym at full speed. If you have no pain,
   d. Do 15 lengths cutting at three-quarter speed. Be sure to plant the outside foot with each cut. If you have no pain,
   e. Do 15 lengths cutting at full speed. If you have no pain,

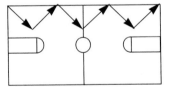

2. Do 10 minutes of running or jumping drills related to your sport. When you have completed the entire program, you are ready to return to competition.*

---

*Each running workout must be followed by a 15-minute application of ice.
†If you do not complete the entire program on a particular day, start at the beginning the following day.

# Index

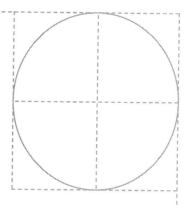

A page number followed by *f* indicates figure; *t* indicates table.